RENDEZVOUS
Pleasing Her

The Tools Men Want for Mastering Non-Sexual & Sexual Skills
for Living The Romantic Lifestyle ...More Fun, Joy, Harmony, Better
Sex and Success in Your Committed Relationship

BENILDA NYA GUERRERO-ORTEGA

authorHOUSE®

AuthorHouse™
1663 Liberty Drive
Bloomington, IN 47403
www.authorhouse.com
Phone: 1-800-839-8640

Published by AuthorHouse 12/17/2012

ISBN: 978-1-4567-6472-2 (sc)
ISBN: 978-1-4567-6473-9 (hc)
ISBN: 978-1-4567-6474-6 (e)

This book is printed on acid-free paper.

Unless otherwise indicated, "Scripture taken from the HOLY BIBLE, NEW
INTERNATIONAL VERSION. Copyright © 1973, 1978, 1984, 1985
International Bible Society. Used by permission of Zondervan Bible Publishers."

How to Order

www.rendezvousexcitinghim.com and rendezvouspleasingher.com

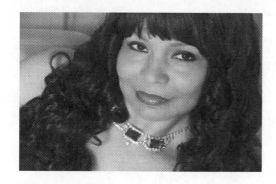

$\mathcal{D}$edication

$\mathcal{T}$o all the couples that are in love and have made a commitment to one another.

$\mathcal{I}$ also dedicate this book to Carlos Ortega; my awesome husband, my partner in life, my confidant and constant encourager. Together, we have braved many storms and our faith, love and mutual respect for each other always helps us persevere. Forever Yours!

Table of Contents

Introduction

With today's wealth of knowledge available on relationship skills, I am delighted that you have chosen to invest in this rendezvous reference book. You have made a winning decision!

I've written this book in honor of marriage, committed relationships and life, and it is written in two convenient versions: "His" and "Hers." These books are chock-full of encouragement, helpful ideas, inspiration and support that interact with each other. I recommend that each of the spouses (your partner in life) have their own version so that you can be assisted and coached simultaneously.

With each Weekly and Daily Coaching you'll find awesome assistance for a happier relationship with your mate and children as well as for your personal and professional life.

I am not suggesting that you become someone that you are not; I'm simply inviting you to stir up your romantic side and develop a new outlook so that you may enjoy the "Forever Pleasure and Excitement" that happen when you give romance the importance that it should have.

How to Use This Book

Take a moment to get acquainted with all that's here so that you can be aware of what's right at your fingertips when you need it. This book will become your journal and rendezvous reference book. It is the type of book that you'll want to carry with you everyday, like your appointment book.

In Part one of this book you'll find knowledge for understanding romance and its basics. There is a place to write her favorite things as well as ideas for romantic quickies, wedding anniversary gifts, ways to celebrate her every month, creative gifts and a suggestion for a very "exciting" night.

Part Two is where the majority of the coaching takes place. It is essential for both of you to be on the same week at the same time so you can carry out the daily coaching practices together.

In Part Three you will be able to continue having fun on a monthly basis as you enjoy yourselves with different ways to take pleasure in monthly holidays and event coaching.

Part Four will assist you in giving and receiving the beautiful gift of Roses and other Flowers with more meaning and gratitude.

Part Five is very important because, you will be able to write more of your mate's favorite things. There will be no more guessing. You will get it right every time and this will show her that you do pay attention, even to the smallest of things.

In Part Six you have space to write all those important dates and contacts, as well as a place to write important notes.

In Part Seven I conclude my coaching by giving you more fuel to fan the flames of Romance with ideas for giving each other pet names, sweet or sexy expressions and how to say "I love you" in other languages as well as the all necessary "Pleasure/Excitement Vouchers."

Throughout this book I have provided space for you to put pictures of your spouse, yourselves and family. I hope this book becomes the essential "Romance Rendezvous Reference" that I intended for it to be – so that you can "forever" please and excite each other and live a happy and victorious life together.

Acknowledgments

I would like to thank the many men and women who took part in my romance research while I was working on this book.

I also want to thank Mary, Max, Celia and Joey whose big heart and dedication helped me in the final organization of the book format.

Additionally, I would like to thank ©Adrian Wilcox Photography for his generosity and great work on my author pictures. Also, Carlos Ortega and Julio Cesar for the photography that was done for this book, as well as the model Einar Soto and Marquita Whittingham for her editing talents.

Finally, I want to thank Virgie Broussard-Pradia, my dance teacher and mentor of many years whose creative writing and excellent talents have inspired hundreds of people. I adore her love for people and passion for life.

$\mathcal{P}$ersonal Data

NAME:_____

ADDRESS:_____

CITY & STATE:_____ZIPCODE:_____

HOME PHONE:_____CELL:_____

E-MAIL:_____

BIRTHDAYS – Spouse:_____Children:_____

WEDDING ANNIVERSARY:_____

FIRST DATE ANNIVERSARY:_____

IN CASE OF EMERGENCY CALL:

NAME:_____Phone:_____

ALLERGIES:_____

MEDICAL ALERTS:_____

BLOOD TYPE:_____

DOCTOR:_____Phone:_____

OTHER SPECIAL EVENTS:

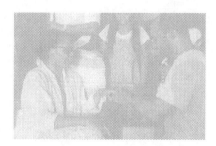

(Place an engagement or wedding picture of the two of you here.)

Part One

Understanding Romance
and
Romance Basics

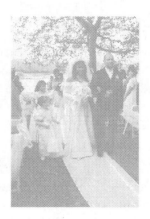

(Place one of your favorite wedding pictures here.)

"Romance"

The word "Romance," awakens different feelings and views in men and women.

Romance… The majority of women, no matter how beautiful and educated, yearn for a man that can understand her need for him to treat her with love, respect and kindness. A man that can help her feel unique and cared for. Someone who can give physical and mental interaction that does not always have to lead to sex.

Romance… For the majority of men, romance means physical and mental interaction that leads to sex, or a fairy-tale world that lives in movies and in novels. Some men and women think that it is something that it's not real or possible, and expensive to achieve.

Most women want and enjoy Non-sexual Romance anywhere and everywhere, but they must have their Sexual Romance as good as it can be… passionate foreplay and tender after-play.

Most men want and enjoy Non-sexual Romance anywhere and everywhere, but they must have their Sexual Romance as good as it can be… hot quickies and passionate lovemaking.

$\mathcal{K}$nowing your mate's emotional state and religious beliefs will help you to appropriately give some thought to how your mate might react to these suggestions before trying them. Your spouse's state of mind and personality will help you to determine whether the attempt is appropriate for your marriage, or even worth the effort. Whatever you do, be sensitive!

$\mathcal{N}$o matter how old you are or how long you've been together, you should create new ways and ideas to surprise your mate.

Benilda Nya

Essentials for Romance

Timing… You want to make sure that your spouse is available for the time you'll need for your display of non-sexual romance or passion for sexual romance. Communication with her will let you know if she has to work late or if it is that time of the month. It will also help you understand her needs: Would she rather stay home and eat take out followed by a foot or full body massage before going to sleep, or eat out followed by dancing—or would she prefer to have time alone? Will she enjoy some hot foreplay followed by a quickie or is she ready for passionate lovemaking?

Setting… The romantic atmosphere must consist of a variety of backdrops: lighting, mood, pleasant aroma, a clean and organized home, favorable conditions as well as some inspiring music. Playing the romantic music that the two of you enjoyed when you were first attracted to each other and started dating, does wonders for renewing that exciting first time feeling. The "Setting," also includes an attractive you: fresh clean and well-groomed body, hands, feet and face (please be careful and don't scratch her with your stubby face). When at home, wear nice or sexy loungewear, and dress nice and sexy when you take her out. Dab on yourself the cologne/fragrance that she loves on you (lightly).

**To produce the best intensity for romance,
the setting must have…**

Passion… The passion for "desiring" and "yearning" someone is a strong force (you were introduced to these feelings when you first fell in love). That passion can create interest and diligence in you to master your touch and foreplay skills, making it incredibly electrifying for her body and soul.

Infuse passion with...

Pleasure... There is a pleasure that goes beyond loving one another. Delighting in each other is vital, taking satisfaction in the mastering of your non-sexual and sexual skills (this is not easy, and it requires daily nourishment). Make a decision to work as hard on your marriage as you do when you put in a 50/60 hour week at work. If you have accomplished great things in your professional life, make sure that you also are proficient in your private life. Take pleasure and pride in creating excellence in your marriage, as well.

Demilla Nyu

Be Her Knight in Shining Armor

*R*omantic heroes know how to set the mood. They take time to explore and to fulfill the Sexual and Non-sexual Romantic desires in the woman they love. Romantic heroes are great lovers because they don't just take pleasure in sex for themselves, but they also enjoy giving pleasure to their woman... serious soul (mind, emotions), spirit & body foreplay.

*Y*ou can create this mood by...

❤ **G**etting rid of all the interruptions ahead of time.

❤ **S**timulating her five senses: soft lighting, comfortable room temperature, silky/soft fabrics, touching her with the right pressure in the places that arouse her, playing sexy music, using sensual aromas, putting on something to please her eyes.

❤ **L**ooking at her with passion and desire: Smile with your eyes, make eye contact look at her when you are going to kiss her or keep looking at her when she is talking to you.

❤ **G**reat kissing: Sensual soft kisses and HOT, Passionate ones, as well.

❤ **U**sing sweet talk/sexy talk: speak with a soft, low voice saying passionate words that let her know how much you want her. Keep the spotlight on her, what you love about her body, how good it feels, the way it smells, and the way it responds to your touch and kisses. Tell her how you want to make love to her. Use words that let her know that you are enjoying every moment with her. Don't talk about past or future things; keep your focus in the present, enjoying the moment. Other sweet talk topics consist of: nature, art, colors, literature, textiles, fashion, food and wine.

Benilda Nya

*M*ake *Way for the Good Habits that Support Romance*

*N*on-sexual Romance is caressing and touching without expectations of a sexual interaction. This is kind of a confirmation of our capability of being concerned about the one we love.

*R*omantic Love is that unbelievable emotion of passion for someone. If you want that feeling to last a lifetime, you need to prevent hurting each other and try to fulfill each other's emotional desires as much as possible. Let's avoid being bankrupted in these areas by successfully making a daily deposit into this account.

*I*t also has to do with you being the leader and the provider. The way a man treats and understands his wife is more important than any physical or material attribute.

A woman wants her husband to respect her, to enjoy loving her "tenderly" and to give her emotional pleasure. You've got to make it good for her.

Benilda Nya

Distrust Will Buy you a One-way Ticket to the Demise of Romance

Do not be a man who is always calling her or getting upset if she does not check in every hour. Do not get upset if she gives another man a compliment. That kind of behavior will destroy your communication and connection and ultimately, her desire for being with you.

If she has done something or continually does things to deserve your distrust then the both of you need to work that out; if necessary, get some counseling. If in the past she did something that she has repented for and has asked you to forgive her, and if she has not violated your trust since, you really should let go of the past so that your future with her can be a peaceful and rewarding one.

Now, if you have been the one to abuse her trust, then you must repent and ask her to forgive you (if you have not already done so). If she is the one checking up on you all the time and you have already mended your ways, then you should have a very serious conversation concerning her trust for you. You need to ask her; "What do you need for me to do to have you trust me?"

There is nothing worse than to live with someone that you can't or don't trust. Without trust it is impossible to have a relationship that is successful and pleasurable. So please, do not abuse and destroy the trust that your wife has in you. To get her to trust in you, you must be consistently honest on a daily basis in every area of your life. Even in the smallest of things, let integrity and excellence be your driving force.

To attract her more, you have to be trustworthy. You should also be able to understand and make provision for her physical, emotional, social, intellectual and spiritual needs. Be kind, patient and supportive and have a loving and positive attitude. Let her know how much you love, respect and value her by treating her like the queen that she is.

Difficult To Romance?

Many married couples have a difficult time being romantic because they do not know how to enjoy each other. Even if they love one another, they just don't seem to have the desire or drive to please and honor each other. Other couple's passion begins to fizzle because of hurt, disappointment or monotony. Either way, they gradually fall apart due to years of, unfulfilled dreams and goals, bitterness or blame.

Other couples become nothing more than business partners who have to maintain their insignificant names ("Mr. and Mrs."), because they do not believe in divorce, or have to stay married because of family, professional, religious or social obligations; counseling maybe of some assistance for these situations.

Some spouses have a physical, mental or medical condition that prevents them from having a fulfilling sexual life with their mate. Please be patient, remember your vows/commitment to this wonderful person, and work on everything possible to find healing and restoration or work together to re-invent your sexual romance.

If you and/or your wife were virgins when you got married, I congratulate you. One of the best things about sexual purity is that you won't be comparing yourselves to anyone else. If you were not virgins, but decided to honor each other by waiting for sexual intimacy until your wedding night, I also congratulate you. It is not easy to have your favorite dessert in front of you and not taste or eat it. Whichever one is your situation, you will have your trials. Please, be patient with her and with yourself as you learn about each other.

In many of these cases my books "RENDEZVOUS - Exciting Him," and "RENDEZVOUS - Pleasing Her," can be a great source of motivation and inspiration to help you and your spouse improve the quality of your marriage. With a positive mental attitude and the desire to improve the quality of your marriage, you can safely navigate to your destination… *Enjoying Each Other and Life Together.*

Benilda Nya

How well do you know her?

*B*y paying attention to her when she speaks and by watching her reactions to things, you will get most of the answers. The rest you will have to get by investigating or by asking her straight out, but please be careful not to give away too much so that you can still keep the element of surprise.

Favorite colors:_____

Type of music she likes:_____

Favorite mood lighting:_____

Favorite travel destinations:_____

Favorite hobbies:_____

Favorite retreat spots/hotels:_____

Surprise ideas:_____

Favorite gift ideas:_____

Favorite precious metals:_____

Favorite plants/herbs/flowers:_____

Favorite precious stones:_____

Favorite perfume/cosmetics:_____

Favorite candle/incense/aromatherapy:_____

Favorite sport(s) & teams:_____

What she likes least about herself/body:_____

_____

Lovemaking positions, places to make love:_____

_____

_____

What can you wear to turn her on:_____

_____

What does she consider romantic or sexy?_____

_____

_____

Favorite place to shop:_____

Clothing & shoe styles/designers:_____

Clothing/shoe size:_____

Favorite accessories:_____

Favorite spa/salon/barber:_____

Favorite toothpaste/soap/shampoo:_____

_____

Favorite books/authors:_____

_____

Best friends:_____

Favorite movies/TV shows:_____

_____

Favorite animals/cartoon:_____

Dream car:_____

Dream house (where, what kind, what would it look like):_____

_____

Favorite Style of Furniture/home accessories:_____

_____

Pet peeves:_____

Things that are embarrassing to her:_____

_____

Favorite TV personality likes/dislike:_____

_____

Favorite influential people:_____

Favorite cologne/fragrance she loves on you:_____

Clothing styles she likes to see you in (for: play, casual, dressy, business):

_____

Things she likes/dislikes about you:_____

_____

Favorite Holiday/time of year:_____

Her work schedule:_____

Where she parks at work:_____

Favorite restaurants:_____

_____

Favorite foods:_____

_____

Favorite desserts:_____

Favorite fruits/nuts:_____

Favorite candies/chocolates:_____

Favorite beverage/wine/champagne:_____

Her worst fear(s):_____

Things she dislikes:_____

Favorite way to relax/de-stress:_____

_____

Other special interests:_____ _____

_____

_____

_____

See page 195– Part Five: for more of her "Favorite Things" to fill in.

Benilda Nya

Romantic Quickies
(Non-sexual)

- **Always walk in to a party, restaurant or special event arm in arm**
- Give her a call during the day just to tell her that you are thinking about her.
- **Tell her: "I love you," or "I'm so in love with you."**
- Make the morning coffee, tea, or juice and bring it to her served on your fine china/crystal.
- **When she's going to sit down to eat at the dinner table pull out her chair for her. Place the napkin in her lap and serve her.**
- Make up the bed in the morning.
- **Before going home, call her and ask her if there is anything she needs from the store.**
- Flirt! Blow her a kiss from across the room. Wink at her. Pinch her softly.
- **Help her get the children ready for school. Or if they are not old enough for school, help her feed them.**
- Do the laundry: wash, dry, fold and put them away where they belong.
- **At night when you are going to sleep, carry her to bed, cover her and kiss her goodnight.**
- On a cold winter night, make some hot cocoa or tea for both of you, cover yourselves with a blanket and cuddle on the couch.
- **On a hot summer day or night, make some lemonade or iced tea and serve it to her.**
- When you are out with her, hold the doors open for her wherever you go.
- **Surprise her with tickets to her favorite event.**
- Open the car door for her, help her in and then close the car door.
- **Help her to keep the house clean or clean the house yourself.**
- Throw out the garbage.
- **Wash her car & put gas in it.**
- Give her a gift for no other reason than just because she is worth it.
- **If you play a musical instrument, play a song for her. Sing to her if you are a singer, write her a song if you write songs.**

ℛomantic Quickies
(Sexual)

WARNING: some may consider some of these suggestions offensive.
Knowing your mate's emotional state and religious believes will help you to *appropriately* give some thought to how your mate might react to these suggestions before trying them. Your spouse's state of mind and personality will help you to determine whether the attempt is appropriate for her, please be sensitive!

- ❤ Give her a call during the day and tell her what you are going to do to her tonight or what you want her to do to you while making love.
- ❤ **Tell her: "I am so turned on by you."**
- ❤ When she's going to sit down to eat at the dinner table (at home) pull out her chair for her. Place the napkin in her lap, caress and kiss her neck then kiss her in the mouth and tell her "you are absolutely delicious." Then serve her dinner.
- ❤ **Before going home call her and ask her if it is possible for her to serve dinner in her high heels and to wear something sexy (provided that she is comfortable and happy doing this).**
- ❤ On a cold winter night, make some hot cocoa or tea for both of you. Cover yourselves with a blanket and, make love on the couch, or on a furry floor carpet by the fireplace.
- ❤ **If you are a good dancer dance for her. Give her a lap dance or just dance sexy to a slow song that she likes.**
- ❤ If you own a swimming pool and have privacy in it: On a hot summer night, make some smoothies, lemonade or iced tea, serve it to her by the swimming pool and go for a skinny dip (please provide for privacy).
- ❤ **When you are out with her, whisper sexy compliments in her ear: "You/your legs look so sexy."**
- ❤ Go to a drive in movie, and while watching the movie take delight in touching and kissing each other.

(As always, please make sure that you have privacy when you want to enjoy some indoor/outdoor sexual romance.)

Benilda Nya

Wedding Anniversary Gifts

	TRADITIONAL	MODERN
FIRST	Paper	Clocks
SECOND	Cotton	China
THIRD	Leather	Crystal/Glass
FOURTH	Fruit/Flowers	Appliances
FIFTH	Wood	Silverware
SIXTH	Candy/Iron	Wood
SEVENTH	Wool/Copper	Desk Sets
EIGHTH	Bronze/Pottery	Linens/Lace
NINTH	Pottery/ Ceramic	Leather
TENTH	Tin/Aluminum	Diamond Jewelry
ELEVENTH	Steel	Fashion Jewelry
TWELFTH	Silk/Linen	Pearls
THIRTEENTH	Lace	Textiles/Fur
FOURTEENTH	Ivory	Gold Jewelry
FIFTEEN	Crystal	Watches
TWENTIETH	China	Platinum
TWENTY-FIFTH	Silver	Silver
THIRTIETH	Pearl	Diamond
THIRTY-FIFTH	Coral	Jade
FORTIETH	Ruby	Ruby
FORTY-FIFTH	Sapphire	Sapphire
FIFTIETH	Gold	Gold
FIFTY-FIFTH	Emerald	Emerald
SIXTIETH	Diamond	Diamond

Please do not forget to give her a card; whether you buy it or whether you make it, the card should never be skipped.

Happy Anniversary Sweetheart

For your Wedding Anniversary, you can be as creative as possible; whether you have fifty dollars, five hundred, five thousand dollars or more (save money for especial occasions), the idea is to make it special, thoughtful and romantically memorable.

Example

For your first wedding anniversary, you can give her a beautiful clock with an inscription like: "Time goes by too slow when I'm away from you." Your husband of one year_____.

Or…

You can take one of her favorite pictures from your wedding and have it made into a 3-D life size poster.

If you are taking her out to dinner for the wedding anniversary, go in style and get the same limousine service that you had for the wedding day (if you did not have a limo service for your wedding, then the anniversary will be a great time to do so). Make the dinner reservation in advance and have the restaurant give you their best private table. Request all white linen, candlelight and either a bottle of her favorite champagne or the brand from the wedding. Arrange with the florist that you used for the wedding to make a replica of the flower centerpiece that you had on your wedding table (any good florist can also do this) or make the wedding bouquet flowers into a centerpiece, and have it delivered to the restaurant to be placed on your table. For dessert, have the baker of your wedding cake replicate two mini-size versions and also have them delivered to the restaurant. Do not skip the anniversary gift; present it to her, during or after your exquisite dinner surprise, beautifully wrapped. (Use your wedding pictures as a guide for the flowers and decorations.)

You can also refer to the back pages of any Bridal magazine to order personalized items like music CD's, champagne/wine bottles etc. What ever you decide to do for the anniversary, do it with thoughtfulness and with serious memories and romance in mind.

Another thing you can do is write the love story of how you met. You could frame it or have it put on a glass or acrylic plaque and give it to her.

Benilda Nya

Be Creative in Your Gift Giving

Take time and effort with the way you wrap and present the gift: use coupons to be redeemed, search and find, follow the trail, hot/cold, solve a mystery, take her out for dinner and have the waiter bring her the gift on a dessert platter. There are also different reasons why you are giving her a gift, and there are many kinds of gifts that you can give to her, for example: A comical gift, Cultural, Spiritual, homemade or custom-made, Inexpensive/Expensive, Sexy/Conservative, Big or Small, Romantic/Practical or to congratulate her on a Social or Professional achievement. You have a lot to choose from, so it does not have to be expected or boring.

For her birthday, give her a gift or surprise her with something really extraordinary each day for the whole birthday month. You can also give her a surprise party like a Hollywood "Red Carpet Event." Have the red carpet and all the photographers (friends with cameras), at the entrance to the banquet hall, club or your house. Videotape it, have someone do the interviews on the red carpet. Get some friends or family members with good taste to help you execute it, or hire an event planner.

Benilda Nya

Every month you have the chance to celebrate her. If she enjoys flowers, give her the flower of the month the first of every month. Give them in different designs and sizes. For her birthday, you could also give her jewelry with her birthstone.

January
Flower: Carnation, Snowdrop
Birthstone: Garnet–constancy
-Celebrating Tip
On the first of January, give her the most beautiful dark red arrangement of carnations and/or Snowdrops she has ever seen.

February - Make this, a Valentine's Month, not just Day
Flower: Violet, Primrose, Begonia
Birthstone: Amethyst–sincerity
-Celebrating Tip
On the first of February, give her a bouquet of Blue Violets. If it's her birthday month and she likes her birthstone, give her jewelry for her birthday.

March
Flower: Daffodil, Jonquil
Birthstone: Aquamarine, Bloodstone–courage
-Celebrating Tip
On the first of March, give her a bouquet of the flower of the month.

April
Flower: Sweet Pea, Daisy
Birthstone: Diamond–innocence
-Celebrating Tip
Give/send assorted colored Daisies or diamond jewelry

May - "Make this a Mother's Day Month"
Flower: Lily of the Valley, Lily
Birthstone: Emerald–love, success
-Celebrating Tip
Give her a bouquet of Lilies of the valley.

June - National Rose Month
Flower: Rose
Birthstone: pearl, alexandrite, moonstone–health

Roses date far back to pre-historic days. They are more than 33 million years old and have been used among friends and lovers to send all sorts of messages, and they are used for many reasons.

-Celebrating Tip
Give her roses every day or week this month. Send or personally give them to her, or place them where she will find them. If she works out of the home, send some to her at work. (Write in the note, card or love letter the meaning of the rose.)

- 💜 *June 1, Give her* **A Crown made of Roses**: *Signifies reward of merit or virtue.*
- 💜 *June 2,* **12 Red and Yellow Roses** *given together: are an expression of congratulations and happy feelings.*
- 💜 *June 3,* **33 Pink Roses**: *"I love you with profound love," Perfect Happiness.*
- 💜 *June 4,* **44 Red & White Roses**: *My vow to you is faithful and consistent; Unchangeable pledge, Unity.*
- 💜 *June 5,* **1 Long Stemmed Red Rose**: *"I will remember you always."*
- 💜 *June 6,* **3 Dark Pink Roses**: *"I love you." "I appreciate you."*
- 💜 *June 7,* **36 Lavender Roses**: *"Reminiscing our romantic time together." I am experiencing romantic affections towards you every time you come near me. Love at first sight.*
- 💜 *June 8,* **A Single Red Rose** *in full bloom: "My love for you is unchanged," or "I still love you."*
- 💜 *June 9,* **9 Red Roses**: *"We'll be together for ever." Eternal love.*
- 💜 *June 10,* **10 White Roses**: *"You are perfect." "You are heavenly."*
- 💜 *June 11,* **11 Light Pink Roses**: *"You are the one I cherish." "You are my treasured one."*
- 💜 *June 12,* **12 Red Roses**: *"Be mine!" Pleasurable combination. Mutual affinity.*
- 💜 *June 13,* **13 Pale Colored Roses**: *"We are for ever friends."*
- 💜 *June 14,* **12 Orange Roses**: *"You are my Fascination." "You Magnetize me."*

- ❤ *June 15,* **40 White and Purple Roses:** *"My love for you is genuine." Symbolic representations of purity and passion.*
- ❤ *June 16,* **2 Coral Roses:** *Two of us deeply in love. Mutual feelings. Enthusiasm. Desire.*
- ❤ *June 17,* **12 Blue Roses:** *"You are extraordinarily wonderful."*
- ❤ *June 18,* **3 Yellow Roses:** *"Its a joy to love you."*
- ❤ *June 19,* **50 Bridal White Roses:** *This is "Regretless/Unconditional Love."*
- ❤ *June 20,* **20 Roses:** *"My feelings towards you are sincere."*
- ❤ *June 21,* **21 Champagne Roses:** *"I'm totally committed to you." "I'm dedicated to you." You are tender and loving.*
- ❤ *June 22,* **Orange and Yellow Roses:** *"Passionate thoughts of you."*
- ❤ *June 23,* **Purple Roses:** *Opulence, Sophistication, Deep magnetism, Greatness.*
- ❤ *June 24,* **24 Red Roses:** *"Forever yours."*
- ❤ *June 25,* **25 Roses:** *"Well done." "Bravo." "Congratulations."*
- ❤ *June 26,* **Pink and White Roses:** *I love you still and always will.*
- ❤ *June 27,* **2 Roses:** *Two of us deeply in love.*
- ❤ *June 28,* **56 Assorted Color Roses:** *"My Love, you're everything to me."*
- ❤ *June 29,* **Green Roses:** *Signifies - Wealth, Constant rebirth of life and energy. Life force, Prosperity. Constant rejuvenation of spirit.*
- ❤ *June 30,* **100 Roses:** *The most pleasurable marriage of the century; we are dedicated to each other forever.*

Famous Rose Quotes

- What's in a name? That which we call a rose/By any other name would smell as sweet. - William Shakespeare, Romeo and Juliet act II, sc. ii
- O, my love's like a red, red rose/That's newly sprung in June. – Robert Burns, A Red, Red Rose
- Rose is a rose is a rose is a rose. – Gertrude Stein, Sacred Emily (1913), a poem well used in Geography and plays.

See Part Four: Flower Meaning (pg 183), for the meaning of the color and story of roses, as well as other flower meanings.

July
Flower: Larkspur, Water Lily, Sunflower
Birthstone: Ruby – contentment
-Celebrating Tip
Have delivered to her a basket of sunflowers or water lilies, or a ruby ring or earrings.

August
Flower: Gladiolus, Poppy
Birthstone: Jade, Peridot, Sardonyx – married, happiness
-Celebrating Tips
1. Bring home or have delivered to her a bouquet of Gladiolus mixed with yellow Poppies
2. Instead of or in addition to flowers: give her Jade, Peridot or Sardonyx jewelry to celebrate your happy marriage.

September
Flower: Aster, Pansy
Birthstone: Sapphire–clear thinking
-Celebrating Tip
Write her a love letter and have it delivered with a bouquet of Asters or Pansies.

October
Flower: Magnolia
Birthstone: Opal, Tourmaline hope
-Celebrating Tip
Give her a flower arrangement of Magnolias, and/or an opal ring.

November
Flower: Chrysanthemum, Orchid
Birthstone: Topaz–fidelity
-Celebrating Tip
Bring/send home a flower arrangement of Orchids.

December
Flower: Hibiscus, Holly, Poinsettia
Birthstone: Turquoise, Zircon - prosperity
-Celebrating Tip
Bring/send home a beautiful Christmas flower arrangement with poinsettias and holly.

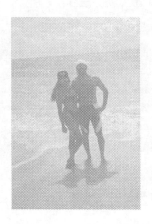

(Place a picture here from when you first met)

Night of Passion (Suggestion for a very "pleasing" night)

(WARNING – some of the language and suggestions contained in the night of passion segment, might be offensive to some.)

Knowing your mate's emotional state and religious believes will help you to appropriately give some thought to how your mate might react to these suggestions before trying them. Your spouse's state of mind and personality will help you to determine whether the attempt is appropriate for her, please be sensitive!

Greet her at the door (whether at home or her favorite hotel suite) by kissing her hand (take her hand and lower you lips to it). Then gently caress her face and lips (if she's wearing lipstick caress above the lip line) and hold her chin up, look into her eyes, tell her how good/ beautiful she looks/is, and kiss her gently but passionately.

Start undressing her at the door, but leave on her under garments and high heels. Carry her into the bathroom where you have prepared a candle lit bubble bath with rose petals in it, her favorite music, fruit, finger food, flowers and beverage (use your fine crystal flute/goblet). Ask her if she wants her hair up, or wrapped in a towel (have some of her hair clips available). After she takes care of how she wants her hair, remove her bra, shoes, then her panties (be gentle), and help her into the bathtub.

Feed her some of the finger food, and then hand her the fine crystal flute/goblet with her favorite drink. After that, feed her some of the fruit. Let her hold on to the glass as you take a sip from your glass and begin to undress yourself (look at her as much as possible during all this) and join her in the tub. Bathe her and have a towel, the food and fruit at hand's reach; and dry your hands and feed her. Repeat this for as long as she wants to keep eating (do not be in a rush). If she wants to bathe you also let her do so, but stay in control, be patient and make it good for her; the evening is still very young.

After a few minutes (20–30) get ready to rinse yourself first, then get out of the tub and dry yourself. Put on your robe or towel. Then rinse her off. Help her up, and dry her with the towel. Dry each foot before it touches the floor mat, and then carry her into the bedroom. The scene there should be a continuation of the ambience from the bathroom: scented candlelight, music, more flowers in the room and rose petals on the bed.

Place her on the bed, kiss her in the mouth passionately, then go into the bathroom and bring out the drinks, the food and fruits, keep the music going. Hand feed her again, and let her drink at her own pace. Start caressing and kissing her all over; face, neck, shoulders, arms, hands/fingers, breasts, belly, hips, legs and feet. Cover all the spots that she wants you to or that you know she likes. (Caress and kiss her breasts not the nipples.)

Then proceed with her favorite lovemaking position. Look directly into her eyes as much as possible. Tell her how incredibly good she feels. Take your time and be passionate. If the position allows; caress and kiss her face and lips. As you caress and kiss her lips, you might want to hold her head up, and if you have whip cream, honey or melted chocolate; dip your finger in it and let her eat it off your finger. Continue kissing her all-over.

Look at the parts you are caressing and kissing. Clasp your hands with hers. Stroke her hair. Grab her hips gently, but with passion. When she does something that pleases you, tell her how good it feels. Whisper sexy things to her (not x-rated), something like; "I love touching you," "You mesmerize me." Create your own, but whatever you say, let it be true, and say it with passion.

After the point of ecstasy has been reached, it is imperative that you spend time in After-play. Snuggle. Cuddle. Take hold of intimacy, and enjoy the present with her. Speak softly, and let her know how much satisfaction she gives you. Fall asleep in each other's arms. And if you wake up in the middle of the night, wake her up gently and whisper to her, "I am so in love with you." In the morning, serve her breakfast in bed (with a flower on the tray). Have food that you know she will enjoy (especially if she's on a diet or eating healthy). Have breakfast in bed with her. Talk to her, tell her how incredible it was and how much you enjoyed her last night. Say only what is true, and say it with passion. If things develop, make love to her again (in bed or in the shower).

Continue for the rest of the day and week touching her in a nonsexual way. Remember: deposits of nonsexual romantic experiences will increase her sexual desire for you.

Plan this according to her schedule. Make sure that she does not have to work late, or that she's not concerned over a project deadline, cleaning the house or that she has the time planned for something else. Call her at work/home (make it quick), and ask her for a date, then carryout your "Night of Passion" for that date. I highly recommend for you to clean the house and/or do the laundry to help ease her duties the day before your date, or you can hire a maid.

If you have children you can plan for a baby sitter, friend or family member to take care of them for about 3-4 hours away from home (if you are staying home), or get an overnight baby sitter if you plan for a night stay at her favorite hotel. Please take caution with burning candles, make sure that they are in the proper containers and away from anything flammable, and that they will last for the time that you need them.

Benilda Nya

Part Two

Pleasurable Weekly and Daily Coaching with Inspirational Sundays

For Monthly Holidays and Event Coaching,
Please See Part Three (page 145).

Select The Current Month, And Agree With Your Mate
To Do The Monthly Coaching Simultaneously.

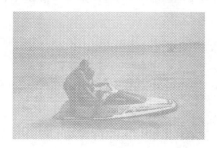

(Place a picture here of both of you doing something fun.)

*D*ecide to fall in love all over again with your mate

. . . .

*I*t takes time to achieve greatness that can last a lifetime

. . . .

*P*ush yourself to greatness because you are lifetime partners

Benilda Nya

He who finds a wife finds what is good and receives favor from the Lord. Proverbs 18: 22 NIV

Say, "I love you" every hour that you are awake, but in a different language each time (see page 218 for saying I love you in other languages).

Stay in tune with your spouse's mood and needs to determine the appropriate romantic approach.

Take her out to lunch or dinner.

Hug her for an extended period of time. (Your goal here is to let her feel protected and loved.)

Let her get frisky.

Give her good morning kisses.

Your physical movement will establish your mental outlook, so head up, shoulders back, stomach in.

Make some hot cocoa or hot tea for the both of you before going to bed. Tell her that you "really" are in love with her. Then make passionate love to her.

Use the pleasure vouchers in the back of this book.

NOTES/COMMENTS/JOURNAL: (Keep a record of what worked, changes made or new ideas.)

Daily Coaching – Week 1

Play Together

On a stormy night, put a puzzle together or play...

Billiards

Dominos

Video Games

Board Games

*P*lay, *P*lay, *P*lay...

Golf

Tennis

Go Bowling

Hide–and Go Seek

Go to the park, ride a seesaw and swing together on the swings.

Benilda Nya

Prepared People Are Ready To Step Into Opportunity.

Sunday

Wise people store up knowledge... Proverbs 10: 14

Monday

Focus on what is good about your mate and marriage.

Tuesday

Call her during the day and tell her that you have everything because you have her.

Wednesday

Flirt with her.

Thursday

Show her passion with your voice.

Friday

Pursue her the way you did when you met her.

Saturday

Do something fun (go to see a play, go skiing or ice skating).

NOTES/COMMENTS/JOURNAL:

Daily Coaching – Week 2

Laughter is Healthy and Necessary in Every Relationship

*S*ome people are naturally playful; they know when to seize the moment to be amusing, while others have to decide to take a chance on the circumstances where humor can take place. A playful person can also make communicating very funny and exhilarating.

I encourage you to play and laugh together because it can be a very healthy factor in the development of a happy relationship. In a stressful moment it can help alleviate the situation and provide emotional relief. The rewards can be tremendous because it can help you to breakthrough the tough times of your relationship. So tickle her act silly, tell her some good jokes or watch a funny movie. If you have kids, include them in on the fun too.

Benilda Nya

If You Have To Debate Within Yourself To Do Right Or Not, You Do Not Have Any Principles.

Sunday

A man/woman who commits adultery lacks judgment; whoever does so destroys themselves and others. Pr. 6: 32 NIV

Monday

Give her passionate kisses. (Be a good kisser.)

Tuesday

Never be a lazy lover; put some energy (more of yourself) into your lovemaking.

Wednesday

Make yourself available for her.

Thursday

Bag the nitpicking.

Friday

Fix breakfast for both of you (and your children), and eat breakfast together.

Saturday

Tell her what it is about her that you love.

NOTES:

Daily Coaching – Week 3

Do you want her to be free and happy in bed?
Encourage Her to be Sexy

If she feels that her body or part of it is not like the way it used to be or like the ones in the magazines or pretty enough, she will tend to shy away from letting you see her completely undressed.

Let her know that she does not need to hide her body from you. More often than not you can help her feel beautiful and sexy. You can cultivate her and be her coach.

With your coaching, she can turn out to be more sexual and free from timidity.

Buy her some nice or sexy loungewear for her to wear around the house (visit my website: BenildaNya.com for store locations).

Praise her!

With your sincere praises, she can become sexier.

Benilda Nya

Nothing Significant Will Happen Until You Take The Initiative.

Sunday

...And the fool multiplies words. No one knows what is coming – who can tell him what will happen? Ecclesiastes 10: 14

Monday

Caress her face, eyes, lips, cheeks, forehead and her hair.

Tuesday

Treat her body like royalty.

Wednesday

Keep your word and promises to her and your children.

Thursday

Tell her that you value her opinion.

Friday

Romantic love is exclusive... Love, laugh, appreciate, understand and strive for excellence in everything you do for your mate.

Saturday

Unconditionally accept each other.

NOTES/COMMENTS/JOURNAL: (Keep a record of what worked, changes made or new ideas.)

Daily Coaching – Week 4

De-stress Together

Boost immunity; live healthier, longer and happier

*M*editate

....

D*o* Tai Chi

....

*P*ractice Qigong

....

*S*tretch together

....

*G*o to your "Happy Place"

....

G*et a manicure & pedicure

....

*D*o deep breathing exercises

....

G*et restored & renewed with a massage

....

*T*ake an aromatherapy bath with lavender oil

....

D*o a 10-minute p.m. yoga de-stressor before going to bed

Benilda Nya

Teach Others How To Love You... Love Yourself.

Sunday

He who gets wisdom loves his own soul... Proverbs 19: 8

Monday

Tell her and show her that you take pleasure in being with her... Have dinner by candlelight.

Tuesday

Touch her in a Non-sexual Romantic way every day, in different ways: in public & in private.

Wednesday

Go to sleep in each other's arms.

Thursday

Let her know how beautiful she is.

Friday

Watch her dress and undress with a sexy lustful smile on your face.

Saturday

Look at her when you are out together. Look at her lips, caress them, and tell her how soft and beautiful and sexy they are.

NOTES:

Daily Coaching – Week 5

43

Do you fantasize coming home and your wife greeting you at the door with: "I want you NOW!"

Flirting with her, will take you to first base; foreplay.

Be careful and exercise self-control and don't just flirt because you want sex. Romance is not a gizmo to negotiate with, but it is a demonstration of your love and honor for her. In order to maximize her desire for sexual romance, it is essential for you to flirt with her everyday.

Benilda Nya

Love Her, The Way She Wants And Needs To Be Loved.

Sunday

What a man/woman desires is unfailing love. Proverbs 19: 22

Monday

Hug her for an extensive period of time (at the movies, watching TV, waiting in lines, at a party or while out with a group of friends).

Tuesday

On a cold winter morning, wrap her up in a warm robe and put warm socks on her (you can warm them up in the dryer). If you have children, you can also do that for them.

Wednesday

Remember your first kiss occasionally and reenact it.

Thursday

Balance your lovemaking style. It shouldn't all be quickies, because you will discourage your mate. And neither should you have to exhaust yourselves in hours of sexual foreplay each time.

Friday

Make your own Romantic scene: kiss as you watch the sunset.

Saturday

Spend the day in bed; read, sleep, play cards/board games. Then take a shower or bath and go back to bed and have dinner in bed (order take-out and have it delivered).

NOTES/COMMENTS/JOURNAL: (Keep a record of what worked, changes made or new ideas.)

Daily Coaching – Week 6

$\mathcal{N}$otice Her

$\mathcal{A}$ woman loves it when the man she loves becomes aware of her physical and intellectual attributes and tells her about them. The incentive to train yourself in this area is that it will do wonders for your sexual romance.

$\mathcal{N}$otice Her Body

$\mathcal{A}$ppreciate the beautiful and pretty parts (be realistic, do not get caught up in the unrealistic, digitally-enhanced version of women's bodies found in Hollywood and magazines). Does she have soft skin, a firm or sexy belly, pretty breasts, tiny waist, nice hips, great looking thighs and legs, well- defined arms, a nice-looking rear end, pretty feet and hands/nails? Is her body in great shape? Does she have a gorgeous looking body? (Whether she is a size 2 or 14, her body can be in great shape, and it can be gorgeous!) Is she wearing something that looks stunning on her? Is the color she's wearing bringing out a dazzling feature of hers? Do you love the way her skin smells?

$\mathcal{I}$f she has gained a few pounds since you met her or since she had the kids, do not criticize and put her down; instead help her to get her shape back by both of you getting on an exercise plan, or by getting a personal trainer for her and by both of you eating healthy (consult with your physician before starting any diet or exercise program).

$\mathcal{N}$otice Her Mind

$\mathcal{N}$otice her ability for problem solving; those great choices and ideas of hers, the flair for home decorating. What are her academic or professional achievements? Compliment and appreciate the way that she connects with you and understands you.

$\mathcal{B}$enilda $\mathcal{N}$ya

When You Love... You Are Happy To Give.

Sunday

He who tends a fig tree will eat its fruit. Proverbs 27: 18

....

Monday

Enjoy kissing all body parts possible. Tell her how sexy and beautiful they are.
You can do this in public (in non sexual ways) and in private.

....

Tuesday

Put her to bed, read to her from a book or story she likes then kiss her
goodnight.

....

Wednesday

After dinner, make some hot chocolate or tea for both of you. Serve it and
cleanup afterwards.

....

Thursday

Makeup the bed in the morning and leave three roses on her pillow.

....

Friday

Make out at the movies and whisper sweet and naughty things to her.

....

Saturday

When she expresses her passion for you, follow along and enjoy.

Use the pleasure vouchers in the back of this book.

NOTES:

Daily Coaching – Week 7

Notice Her Hair

*D*id she just get a new style, cut, color? Is her hair shiny and healthy looking? Does it smell good? Does she have beautiful curls? Is her hair beautifully straight? Does it fall in a special way on her face, neck or shoulders. Do you like the way it feels?

*V*erbalize it!

*W*hat about her face? Her smile, her pretty/soft skin, bone structure, eyes, lips, teeth, eyebrows, nose, eyelashes, makeup.

*T*he way she talks, walks, sits, eats, drinks, crosses her legs…is it sexy? Express what "truly" excites you about her.

*T*ell Her!

*I*s she a good housekeeper, good cook, neat, do you like the way she takes care of you and the kids? Does she do a great job with the laundry/ironing? Did she do or buy something new for the house to make it more beautiful?

Get her fully acquainted with how unique and priceless she is to you.

With a woman there is always something that a man can compliment. Some of these flattering remarks do not need to be said but once or twice a month. No one likes to be taken for granted!

If you feel like there are not too many good things to notice about her, think again. Could it be stress, the children, an unaccomplished goal or dream. Has something happened in the relationship to take away your interest? What was it about her that attracted you when you first met her? If she has lost some of that sparkle, find out what you can do to help her get it back.

Benilda Nya

Sunday

Love is patient, love is kind. It does not envy, it does not boast, it is not proud. It is not rude, it is not self seeking, it is not easily angered, it keeps no record of wrongs. Love does not delight in evil but rejoices with the truth. It always protects, always trusts, always hopes, always perseveres. 1 Corinthians 13: 4-7

Monday

Exercise together.

Tuesday

Buy her a new outfit (make sure it is a style and color that she loves).

Wednesday

Wake up before her and make her her favorite breakfast.

Thursday

Call her during the day to see how she is doing.

Friday

Light some aromatherapy candles, play relaxing music and debrief together from the stresses of the week: stretch and breathe in deeply.

Saturday

Feed each other while making love. Share chocolates, fruits or chocolate covered fruits with champagne or your favorite beverage in a hot tub or in bed.

This is particularly great if you want to play a Greek night fantasy, or a Cleopatra and Anthony Egyptian night. With this beautiful world that God created with its vast selection of cultures, there are so many themes to choose from for sexual romance: Choose a different culture or Country every month to inspire your lovemaking.

NOTES/COMMENTS/JOURNAL: (Keep a record of what worked, changes made or new ideas.)

Daily Coaching – Week 8

❤ *G*ive her the confidence needed to look her best.

❤ *W*hen other attractive women are around, tell your wife: "you are gorgeous."

❤ *W*hen you take her out, persuade her to dress in the sexy, stylish and classy clothes that fit her fashion personality and body type.

Benilda Nya

How Do You Feel/Think About Yourself?... You Are The Way You See Or Think About Yourself.

Sunday

As water reflects a face, so a man's heart reflects the man. Proverbs 27: 19

Monday

Praise her for her great household skills and help her keep the house clean, beautiful and inviting.

Tuesday

If she looks good dressed up for work, tell her.

Wednesday

Join her in playing the music that helps both of you relax, and take an aromatherapy bath together.

Thursday

Realize the importance of good, sexual romance so that you can keep your wife craving for you.

Friday

After dinner, make some hot chocolate or tea, serve it. Then cuddle and talk and/or listen to music.

Saturday

Break out the bubbly for dinner.

Keep a good stock of wine and champagne in your house (replace with alcohol free if you don't do liquor).

NOTES:

Daily Coaching – Week 9

Getting To Know Her

Is she...

Sad

Sick

Bored

Hungry

Worried

Fatigued

Overloaded

Overwhelmed

Does she have Low Self Esteem?

Arguments or discontent tend to increase rapidly when one of these physical and mental factors is present. Becoming aware of these issues will help you to be especially sensitive about what her needs are and how you speak to her and what you talk to her about. It will also give you insight on how to listen to her, and help you to understand her state of mind.

You can also help her by finding a way to alleviate the problem. You might need to give her time alone, or she might need some extra nurturing, pampering or maybe even a pep talk. (Take care of her.)

Wisdom in the basic skills of communication, conversation and relationships will help you choose the emotional ambiance you would like in your relationship and in your home.

Benilda Nya

Be A Man Of EXCELLENCE!

Sunday

A man is praised according to his wisdom, but men with warped minds are despised. Pr. 12: 8 NIV

Monday

Flirt with her over the phone

Tuesday

Tell her that she is your life coach.

Wednesday

Empower yourself; learn to be a great lover. Learn what to do to her body by exploring it and asking her what she likes.

Thursday

Clean up the kitchen after dinner (the way she likes it), then cuddle and talk and/or listen to music.

Friday

Be willing and ready for a surprise.

Saturday

After dinner, put on some slow love songs and very passionately dance with her and tell her how much you love her.

NOTES/COMMENTS/JOURNAL: (Keep a record of what worked, changes made or new ideas.)

Daily Coaching – Week 10

Getting to Know You

*A*re you...

Sad

Sick

Bored

Hungry

Fatigued

Overloaded

Overwhelmed

Do you have Low Self Esteem?

*A*rguments or discontent tend to increase rapidly when one of these physical and mental factors is present. Become aware of these issues and help her to understand your needs, so that she can be especially sensitive and comprehend your mood and if possible fulfill your desires. You can give her insight on how to lend a hand and assist you in a quick recovery.

Benilda Nya

SUCCESS Only Comes Before Work In The Dictionary.

Sunday

He who works his land will have abundant food. Proverbs 12: 11

Monday

Share her excitement in the things that excite her.

Tuesday

Meet her for lunch.

Wednesday

Honor her by listening to what she has to say and understand her.

Express your feelings about something that is bothering you (in a respectful, non-condemning way).

Thursday

Tell her that she's the one that you just can't live without!

Friday

Thank her for understanding you.

Saturday

Show your gratitude; take her shopping for a pair of new shoes and purse at her favorite store.

NOTES:

Daily Coaching – Week 11

*G*o out on a date at least once a week. Have fun the way you used to when you were dating.

(If you have children, plan for this according to their ages.)

Benilda Nya

Do What Is Right Even If No One Is Watching.

Sunday

The man of integrity walks securely, but he who takes crooked paths will be found out. Proverbs 10: 9

Monday

Play as hard as you work.

Tuesday

Become masterful in the bedroom. Excel in all areas of manhood. Do not use sex to control your mate, use sex to serve her and to give her and yourself pleasure. Do it well!

Wednesday

Encourage her beauty, her good ideas, her feelings, creativity, intelligence and opinions. By doing this, you will express your love for her.

Thursday

Carry her to bed.

Friday

Make time for her to pamper you.

Saturday

Give her the day off. Drop her off/send her to her favorite spa/salon for a complete or partial overhaul. (Make the appointment and plan for this according to your budget.)

NOTES/COMMENTS/JOURNAL: (Keep a record of what worked, changes made or new ideas.)

Daily Coaching – Week 12

*M*arriage will challenge your ability to be resilient; it will dare your imagination to come up with positive resolutions. For a successful marriage, sometimes you will need to put your mate's satisfaction before your own. The denial of self is a great way to convey your love for your spouse.

*A*s you nurture your relationship, be independently strong as you also depend on each other for certain things.

*T*he bonds of holy matrimony sometimes entail pain and struggle, and the restraint and effort that are analogous to our pedagogical and professional development. But it is also rewarded with the satisfaction of achieving your goals and making your dreams a reality.

*S*o go ahead and walk that extra mile and do those special things for your spouse, the reward of "absolute pleasure" is well worth it.

Benilda Nya

"Most Folks Are About As Happy As They Make Up Their Minds To Be."
– Abraham Lincoln

Sunday

For as he thinketh in his heart, so is he... Proverbs 23: 7

onday

Round out your rough edges.

Tuesday

Give her a bubble bath, and wash her hair.

Wednesday

Tell her; "I am so in love with you."

Thursday

Give her "sweet" good morning kisses.

Friday

Surprise her with 2 or 3 movie tickets for her to go see a movie with her friends.

Saturday

Make breakfast for the both of you, serve her and yourself, and eat breakfast in bed.

NOTES:

Daily Coaching – Week 13

*A*bsolute pleasure also comes through the recognition, love and encouragement of your spouse. Do not be possessive or consider yourself the most important part of the marriage relationship. Leave the past behind; do not let it determine your future. Initiate what you want out of your marriage. Learn to celebrate your spouse instead of just tolerating her. Show her that your love has no restrictions to its staying power and no end to its hope; your love for her will survive everything!

(For your safety and well-being in relationships where there is abuse, addictions or mental problems: no restrictions to staying power and hope, need to be re-evaluated.)

Benilda Nya

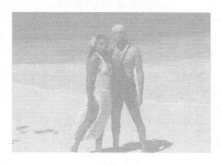

(Place a picture of the both of you here.)

Write down your goals and go over them daily. Take 2 - 3 minutes and see yourself accomplishing them and feel the way you will when they come to pass. This will increase your chances for achievement by more than 90%.

Sunday

Then the Lord replied: "Write down your vision, and make it plain on tables (paper), that he may run that readeth it. Habakkuk 2: 2

Monday

Be consumed with her strengths.

Tuesday

Take advantage of her erotic possibilities; touch, caress and kiss her skin.

Wednesday

Cherish her. Think highly of her and tell her that you think highly of her.

Thursday

Kiss her, hug her and tell her that she is amazing and beautiful.

Friday

Take her out for dinner at a four-or five-star restaurant. Make good use of social and table etiquette.

Saturday

Take a motivational class together to increase your level of excitement in everything you do.

Use the pleasure vouchers in the back of this book.

NOTES/COMMENTS/JOURNAL: (Keep a record of what worked, changes made or new ideas.)

Daily Coaching – Week 14

While making love, tell her how much you want her.

Benilda Nya

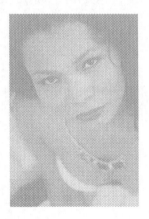

(Place a sexy picture of her here.)

Choices = Results… Please Do Not Make A Permanent Choice In A Short-Lived Situation.

Sunday

Like a bird that strays from its nest, is a man who strays from his home. Proverbs 27: 8 NIV

Monday

Call her during the day and flirt with her.

Tuesday

Make time to listen to her and be considerate of the way she feels.

Wednesday

Value her… Put her to sleep with a relaxing back-massage.

Thursday

Develop self-discipline, increase in knowledge regularly and expand your vocabulary.

Friday

Appreciate the way that she shows her love for you.

Saturday

Surprise her with tickets to a concert or the opera. Dress handsomely according to the event, and treat her as royalty.

NOTES:

Daily Coaching – Week 15

What is it about her that turns you on?

Tell her.

Benilda Nya

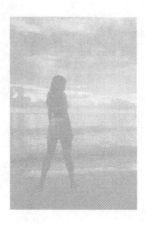

(Place another sexy picture of her here.)

Be RELENTLESS… When It Comes To Accomplishing Your Dreams, Goals, Purpose, Destiny And Your Happiness.

Sunday

A cheerful heart is good medicine, but a crushed spirit dries up the bones. Proverbs 17: 22

Monday

Believe in yourself. Focus on achieving your goals.

Tuesday

Give her "delicious" good morning kisses.

Wednesday

Rekindle your desire and passion for your wife.

Thursday

Be open to her suggestions.

Friday

Take her out dancing.

Saturday

Be ready, willing and thankful for TLC.

NOTES/COMMENTS/JOURNAL: (Keep a record of what worked, changes made or new ideas.)

Daily Coaching – Week 16

All About the Family

If you have children, you should develop a good relationship with them. You can play with them and depending on their age, teach them a game or sport. You could also take golf or tennis lessons together as a family. Maybe you can do a craft project or build something together.

Start this relationship when they're little so that you can have a better chance at those possibly trying teenage years.

The benefits are enormous because not only will you encourage and give your children the emotional and spiritual support that is essential for them to have, but you and your mate can also get pleasure from acting like kids again thus strengthening your romantic relations.

Teach your kids from an early age to be appreciative and thoughtful. Teach family values; encourage them to give gifts and cards to you, your wife, family and friends. They can design and make the cards and gifts or if they have a talent, encourage them to; write and sing a song, choreograph a dance, play their instrument, paint a picture or write a poem, etc.

Instruct and help your teenagers with their self-respect and help them with their self-esteem. Train your children to be self-sufficient and how to protect themselves and what to do in case of an emergency.

To understand each other's temperament better and to improve your communications, I recommend that you and your family take a test to find out the "personality type" of each of you.

Benilda Nya

Parents Are The Stage And Inspiration, For Their Children To Create On.

Sunday

Train a child in the way he should go, and when he is old he will not turn from it. Proverbs 22: 6

Monday

Why don't you and the kids wake Mom up with kisses?
Before you go to sleep, think of at least 3 things that you are happy about, and thank God for them.

Tuesday

Take her out to lunch.
Get the kids ready for tomorrow for her.

Wednesday

Make time for eating breakfast together as a family.
Call her during the day just to tell her that you LOVE her.

Thursday

Wakeup up grateful! Think of 3 things to be thankful for.
Put a pink rose on her pillow before she goes to bed.

Friday

Do the laundry just the way she likes it; if the kids are old enough let them help you.

Saturday

Let her be free to express her femininity, enjoy and encourage it.
Find out if she is available next Saturday, then, make an appointment for her at her favorite Spa, to get a facial and/or massage, manicure and pedicure. Then let her know that you need her for a couple of hours on that day, without giving the surprise away. Arrange for her transportation: you can drop her off and pick her up or hire a Limo service or Taxi. The day of her surprise, serve her breakfast in bed and make sure that she is on time for her pampering. While she is at the Spa, you can clean the house and prepare or order a late lunch/early dinner. When she gets back, set the table and serve the meal, cleanup afterwards.

Daily Coaching – Week 17

Is She A Mom?

Creating romantic moments takes on a whole new meaning when you have children. Your wife will need a little more TLC from you, and you will need a lot of patience. The children should be taught discipline and consideration from day one so that they can understand the need for Mom and Dad to have time alone. Do not hesitate to display *non-sexual romance* in front of your children. This will create a sense of security for the family: your boys will learn to be romantic, and the girls will appreciate and look for a man who will treat them well and is romantic. This will also help them in selecting a good mate and in having a successful relationship.

- ❤ The family should spend quality time together.
- ❤ The children will grow up and make a life for themselves, so make sure that you nurture your marriage with romance if you still want to have one after they leave.
- ❤ Give them (each of your children and your wife) your undivided attention, and tell them that you love them.
- ❤ You and your wife should agree on how to raise and discipline the children (never disagree on the method of discipline in front of the children).

Benilda Nya

Do Not Criticize Your Spouse Or Child Constantly. Instead Use The: "Positive" – "Negative" – "Positive" Method.

Sunday

He who heeds discipline shows the way to life, but whoever ignores correction leads others astray. Proverbs 10: 17

Monday

Before leaving for work, group hug with the kids and wife, kiss them and tell them how much you LOVE them.

Tuesday

Always kiss her goodnight.

Wednesday

Get the kids ready for tomorrow for her.

Thursday

It's a beautiful life. (You get what you say, what are you saying?)
Dress nice for dinner with Benilda Nya's "Loungewear Home-line" for men.

Friday

Help her to cleanup after dinner.

Saturday

If you were able to schedule her for some spa time, serve her breakfast in bed and tell her about the surprise you have for her. (If you were not able to give her the spa time, serve her breakfast in bed and prepare her a soothing bubble bath.)

Plan a homemade costume dinner party just for you guys. If you have children and they are old enough, get them involved too, and give away prizes for best costume, best creativity, color, etc (first, second, third, fourth, fifth place). Just make sure every body gets a prize. Let your child/kids decide which award goes to Mom and Dad. Put your child/kids to bed, and then… appreciate and enjoy her spontaneity and creativity for sexual romance.

Daily Coaching – Week 18

If you are a father, teach your children from a young age to be courteous and romantic.

❤ Teach your boy(s) how to give genuine compliments to their Mother, sister, grandmothers, aunties and to their girl cousins. Instruct him/them on good manners, and social etiquette skills: to open doors and hold doors open for the ladies; to pull the dinner chair out if she is getting up, or push the chair in when she is sitting down, and to give a hand in carrying a shopping or grocery bag. Teach him/them to be neat and to help around the house. (He/they will also learn by watching you do these things.) Thank your child for being trustworthy and well behaved. Tell him "I love you," and how handsome he is.

❤ Romance your daughter(s): Bring/send her, her favorite flowers. Compliment her: beautiful hair, pretty face, hands, dress, etc. Tell her that you love her, and that she is beautiful and smart. If she behaves well, tell her. Display good manners: hold the door open, pull/push the chair; use your social etiquette skills. Thank her for being trustworthy. Be attentive to her needs and wants.

(Do this according to the age of your child.)

Benilda Nya

Discipline your son, and he will give you peace; he will bring delight to your soul. Proverbs 29: 17

The righteous man leads a blameless life; blessed are his children after him. Proverbs 20: 7

Your Attitude Makes A Big Difference.

Sunday

Everybody pitch in and cook a BIG breakfast: cook everybody's favorite food including those foods from your native Country (if other than American). Everyone also contributes in the clean up.

Better to live in a desert than with a quarrelsome and ill-tempered mate. Proverbs 21: 19

Monday

Go out for breakfast.
Before she goes to sleep, kiss her and tell her that you LOVE her.

Tuesday

Get the kids ready for school.
Put her to bed and read her a story, or read from her favorite book.

Wednesday

Help out with the laundry, and do it the way she likes.

Thursday

When she asks you for help, make yourself available to her and help her.

Friday

Take time out to enjoy each other!

Saturday

Give her the day off.

Start the morning by playing her favorite songs as you and the kids (if any) make breakfast and start the Saturday chores. When you are finished, take your child/kids to a movie or their favorite game room, park or simply rent some movies, make some popcorn and have fun lounging around the house.

NOTES:

If you are a father, teach your children from a young age to be courteous and romantic.

❤ Enroll your children in etiquette classes; it will be one of the best investments that you can ever make for their future, (please make sure that you also practice your manners with them and around them; be the example). Teach them to respect others and how to deal with difficult people. Do not spoil your children; you will just make it hard for them to succeed in life and function well in society.

❤ Remember that you and your wife are the ones that have the power to instill and create in your child/children the basic ingredients for a successful life. They are like a blank tape ready to record, therefore *you* greatly determine their values and character along with the social environment that you expose them to. Develop trust, learn to communicate well with your child/children and be an inspiration.

(Do this according to the age of your children.)

Benilda Nya

A good man/parent leaves an inheritance for his children's children. Proverbs 13: 22

Be very careful with the behavior that you accept from your child because, that is the behavior that you approve of.

Sunday

Folly is bound up in the heart of child, but wise discipline and correction will drive it far from him. Proverbs 22: 15

Monday

Kiss and hug and wish her a great day before leaving (if you have kids include them in also).
Get the children's clothes ready for tomorrow. Put the kids to bed.

Tuesday

Pay attention to details.
Kiss your wife hello first then the kids and group hug. Ask how their day was.

Wednesday

Let your wife know that she won't need to cook tonight.
Bring dinner and dessert home.

Thursday

Make sure the kid's homework is done right, and then let her ask everybody (including you) to pickup a good book and read a couple of chapters.

Friday

Make a healthy breakfast for your self & your wife/family.
Take a walk hand in hand or go for a drive after dinner & tell your wife that you'd rather be with her right there than any other place in the world. (Feel it & mean it.)

Saturday

Give your wife a non-sexual bath (prepare a bubble bath and play her favorite music).

NOTES/COMMENTS/JOURNAL: (Keep a record of what worked, changes made or new ideas.)

Daily Coaching – Week 20

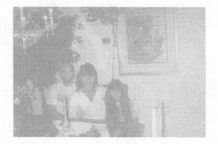

(Place your family picture here.)

Write Down Five Things That You Are Grateful For

1.

2.

3.

4.

5.

Think About These; Every Morning As Soon
As You Wakeup & Give Thanks.

To look the very best that you can look... Stay in Shape

*G*et a good night's sleep

....

Exercise three to five times a week

....

*E*at healthy and drink plenty of good water

....

For good health, stay within the desired weight for your height

....

*E*xercise your brain (learn a new hobby, work on word or picture puzzles)

....

This regimen is great for anti-aging.

Take care of yourself; she needs you around for a long time, and she needs you to function well in spirit, body and soul.

(Consult with your doctor before beginning any form of diet and exercise.)

Benilda Nya

Connecting With Wise People Will Stimulate Your Imagination.

Sunday

He who walks with the wise grows wise, but a companion of fools suffers harm. Proverbs 13: 20

Monday

Be Passionate about pleasing her!

Tuesday

Share your feelings openly instead of shutting down or quarreling.

Wednesday

Don't forget to help out with the morning house chores.

Thursday

Devotion is essential for success. Devote yourself to your marriage.

Friday

Part of being a great husband is to also be a great lover.

Saturday

Do not let her anticipate your moves; do something new to her, something totally unexpected.

NOTES:

Daily Coaching – Week 21

$\mathcal{A}$t the end of the day, both of you will need to recover from your day. Give yourselves at least thirty minutes to an hour to refresh and renew your spirit, body and soul. Talk it over with her to decide who goes first. Be kind. If you both need the same time off, then rotate and respect that time.

....

$\mathcal{S}$tart a book club. Take the family (spouse and children if old enough) to your favorite bookstore and find a book of your choice. Buy everybody his or her own book if you can. Designate a night during the week or weekend when everybody can take an hour or so to read their book (great family reading time). You can have your favorite dessert and beverages while you read (if you have only one book, you can rotate reading to each other).

Once a week over dinner you can discuss each chapter as it ends, until the book is finished. As you start a new book let another family member choose the next book. (You can also do this just with your wife and other family members as well as with friends or neighbors.)

Benilda Nya

BE FAITHFUL!

Cater to your woman.

Drink water from your own cistern (container), running water from your own well. Proverbs 5: 15

Make a healthy breakfast for your self & your wife/family.

Call her during the day and ask her to order dinner from her favorite restaurant. Have it delivered or you can pick it up on the way home.

Hug her around her waist and with a whisper tell her in her ear how irresistible she is.

Be uncomplicated to love.

Let your soft kisses wake her up in the morning.

Always accept her invitation. Make sure that you look good for that date, use your good manners, give her a rose or a small thank you gift, and enjoy.

NOTES/COMMENTS/JOURNAL: (Keep a record of what worked, changes made or new ideas.)

Daily Coaching – Week 22

Exciting Things to Do Under the Full Moon

❤ Take a few minutes together to gaze at the moon if it is in view and share some romantic thoughts.

❤ Take her to the beach to watch the full moon rise; hold her hand and recite a romantic poem to her, then kiss her hand softly and passionately on her lips.

❤ If the weather permits have a candle lit dinner in the backyard or balcony under the moonlight.

❤ Take her on a dinner cruise. As you watch the full moon hug her from behind, lean your head on hers and whisper "I am so in love with you," talk of sweet and romantic things (be sincere). Kiss and caress her.

❤ Take her out on your boat, or rent a yacht for the evening.

❤ Go for an evening stroll arm in arm, around the neighborhood or local park.

❤ If you have your own private swimming pool, go skinny-dipping and make love to her in the pool.

❤ Make passionate love to her under the moon light. (Make her quiver with pleasure… Give her a "G" spot orgasm.)
(As always, please provide for privacy when engaging in outdoor sexual romance.)

Benilda Nya

Choose To Disagree Nicely.

Sunday

Allow yourself to be pampered, and when she suggests that you take the day off; do something you enjoy doing or just lounge around the house and do nothing.

Better to live on a corner of the roof than share a house with a quarrelsome wife. Proverbs 23: 24

Monday

Wake up counting your blessings; have a happy day!

Tuesday

Make a vision board of your accomplishments.

Wednesday

Have dinner out in your yard, balcony or at the beach.

Thursday

Get rid of procrastination.

Friday

If you have kids you could think about having a family talent show night.

Saturday

Bathe each other in an aromatherapy bubble bath. Light some candles, play some music and have your favorite beverage.

NOTES:

Daily Coaching – Week 23

Make Her Feel Like a Woman Should

*M*ost women enjoy seeing the expression in their man's eyes when they are being made love to. So look at her, talk sexy or make sexy sounds to express your pleasure, let her be the center of your attention. Caress her lips, face and body while making love. Let your mouth, arms and hands show her how much you enjoy her body. Take your time, do it with passion.

Benilda Nya

You Might Not Be Able To Control The Circumstances, But You Definitely Can Control The Way You React.

Sunday

A wise man has great power, and a man of knowledge increases strength. Proverbs 24: 5

Monday

Stay in tune with your spouse's mood and needs to determine the appropriate romantic approach.

Tuesday

Make breakfast.
Go out for an evening stroll.

Wednesday

Decide to succeed.

Thursday

Call her during the day and tell her that you have everything because you have her.

Friday

After dinner, go count the stars and watch for falling stars to wish upon.

Saturday

Spend the whole day in bed: reading, eating, talking, watching movies, etc.

NOTES/COMMENTS/JOURNAL: (Keep a record of what worked, changes made or new ideas.)

Daily Coaching – Week 24

WARNING – some of the language and suggestions contained below, might be offensive to some.

Pleasure & Excitement

*S*exually arousing her will take some desire, know how and effort.

- ♥ What is the mood that makes her most receptive to or eager for sex?
- ♥ How can you dress to turn her on?
- ♥ What helps her to loosen up and get into you?
- ♥ What type of lighting does she like?
- ♥ Are you a good kisser?
- ♥ Do you smell the way she likes?
- ♥ Does she like a sensual massage? Do you know how to give her one?
- ♥ What type of music puts her in the mood?
- ♥ Will satin bed sheets make it more erotic for her?
- ♥ Are there any adult toys that she would enjoy?
- ♥ What are her favorites on the foreplay menu?
- ♥ Take time out for after-play. How does she like her after-play?
- ♥ In what places is she most open to make love or have sex?
- ♥ What sexual positions does she like?
- ♥ Let her concentrate on the sensations that you want to provoke in her by you being the giver (do this at least once a month).

Benilda Nya

Be At Peace And Have Faith, While You Are Working To Achieve Your Dreams And Goals. They Will Happen!

Sunday

A heart at peace gives life to the body but envy rots the bones. Proverbs 14: 30

Monday

Make your dreams a reality by concentrating on the details.

Tuesday

Be confident, think well of yourself and believe in yourself.

Wednesday

Let her know that you are taking care of dinner tonight.
Cook or bring home dinner and cleanup afterwards.

Thursday

Whenever she wants to EXCITE you sexually, free your mind and enjoy!

Friday

Go ahead and share a piece of string licorice or gum without using your hands.

Saturday

Have breakfast in the backyard or on the porch or balcony.

NOTES:

Daily Coaching – Week 25

Be Her #1 Fan

*A*ward your spouse with a plaque or trophy (make it big and/or beautiful) for being "The Greatest" or "Best" _____, or for a professional, sporting or hobby accomplishment. Plan an awards dinner, invite family, friends, co-workers and especially the people that appreciate and respect her and are a part of the group concerning this award. You can send out invitations and make the party or dinner casual, semi-formal or formal according to the type of award.

*Y*ou could make it a surprise; just make sure that she is available for that day by asking her for a date or you could just tell her that a party/dinner is being held in her honor. Let her know how she needs to dress. You could buy her a new outfit; send her to the beauty salon to get her hair done as well as a manicure and pedicure. Make sure that she looks beautiful.

*S*elect some of these happy supporters to say a few words and make the presentation speech a real good one. You can hold this party/dinner at her favorite restaurant, venue or at home.

*Y*ou could make the party be like a red carpet event; the red carpet at the entry, a couple of photographers taking pictures and a couple of video cameras filming the event as well as interviewing the guests on their well wishes for the honoree. Every body should be wearing their best for this one. You could hire a party planner to help you execute this event.

Benilda Nya

Weekly Coaching - Week 26

Develop And Refine Yourself.

Sunday

My son, preserve sound judgment and discernment, do not let them out of your sight; they will be life for you. Proverbs 3: 21-22

Monday

Hello and goodbye kisses are always a delight.

Tuesday

Separate yourself from the people and things that will hinder your success.

Wednesday

Make a fruit salad for dessert and feed her and yourself.

Thursday

Touch her in non-sexual romantic way.

Friday

Look and feel sexy. Have a great loungewear home-line and pajama arsenal. Use them daily.

Saturday

Take her to the beach for a picnic dinner, and watch the sunset while hugging her and whispering sweet nothings to her.

NOTES/COMMENTS/JOURNAL: (Keep a record of what worked, changes made or new ideas.)

Daily Coaching – Week 26

*L*et Her Know that you Treasure Being with Her

❤ Make time for her.

❤ Hug her for an extensive period of time.

❤ Hug her at the movies, as you're waiting in line, at a party or while out with a group of friends.

❤ Hug, kiss and caress her; whisper sweet words of love to her after making love.

❤ Walk hand in hand, arm in arm or with arms around each other.

❤ Let her know how much you miss her: when you go away on a business, trip arrange with your jeweler to deliver to her a jewelry gift with a romantic note or inscription.

❤ Get to know her so well that just by her looking at you or you looking at her in certain situations you know what she wants or feels.

❤ Respect her, and try to understand her frame of mind.

❤ Give her some space, time to herself and time with her friends.

Benilda Nya

Your Most Powerful Tool And Weapon Is YOUR Mouth. Use It Responsibly.

Sunday

The tongue has the power of life and death, and those who love it will eat of its fruit. Proverbs 18: 21

Monday

Learn a new language together.

Tuesday

Praise her for her uniqueness.

Wednesday

Until you decide to do it, it's not going to happen.

Thursday

Do some "Pillow" talk.

Friday

Enjoy her sexual flirtations.

Saturday

Take her to see a play, a concert, the ballet or an opera. Let her know in advance so that she can dress appropriately. Make sure that you also dress for the occasion, look and smell good, and please don't forget to use good social etiquette.

NOTES:

Daily Coaching – Week 27

Look Your Best

DRESS FOR SUCCESS

*Y*our success will depend a lot on your appearance, communication skills (verbal/non-verbal) and business etiquette. Have the right attitude at work and for work.

DRESS SEXY/STYLISH (When You Go Out with Her)

*U*se the right colors and trendy or classic styles to go with your fashion personality and body type. Make sure that the clothes are clean, pressed, fit properly and are neatly in place. Make sure that there are no split seams, hanging threads, sagging linings or loose buttons. Your shoes should also be clean and polished with no worn heels and free of bad odors. Under garments should be as new. No holes, stains or worn out.

BE WELL-GROOMED (To guarantee your good looks.)

<u>Hair</u> - Your style should be an updated look that you can style and keep looking good between visits to the barber, and it should be a style that goes with the shape of your face. If you color your hair or put highlights in it, make sure you keep up with the retouching. **Facial hair** - Can affect your image (depending on your profession, you should stay away from facial hair). It should be well-trimmed and not overstated. **Your face** - Use the right products for your skin type; they will keep your skin looking good. (Go for a facial at least once a year.) **Eyebrows** - Bushy eyebrows are not too attractive, so please have them trimmed. <u>Clip</u> those unsightly ear and nose hairs. <u>If you wear eye glasses</u>, wear the right color and shape for your face or get contacts; you can also try to see if laser eye surgery is for you. **Mouth** - Brush & floss daily. Make sure that your breath is fresh. If you have problem or damaged teeth, you can improve their appearance by bleaching, bonding, porcelain veneers or crowns. **Body** - Bathe daily. Keep yourself nice and fresh (clean smelling from head to toes); after all, you might get a surprise treat from your wife. Dab on your/her favorite cologne or aftershave (lightly please).

Benilda Nya

Success Requires Knowledge.

Sunday

Take her to a museum or art gallery.

It is not good to have zeal without knowledge, nor to be hasty and miss the way. Proverbs 19:2

Monday

Get rid of nagging habits.

Tuesday

Celebrate her beauty.

Wednesday

Call her during the day to see how she's doing; ask if she needs anything brought home tonight.

Thursday

Be committed to self-discipline.

Friday

Cuddle after dinner.

Saturday

Take time to relax, talk and listen to each other about any concerns, or plans for something.

NOTES/COMMENTS/JOURNAL: (Keep a record of what worked, changes made or new ideas.)

Daily Coaching — Week 28

Look Your Best/Be Your Best

BE WELL-GROOMED (To guarantee your good looks.)
<u>Fingernails</u> - should be clean and filed with trimmed cuticles. (Get a manicure and pedicure at least once a month.) Use a pumice stone on your hands a couple of times a week to control roughness. **<u>Manscaping/Body Grooming</u>** - trim, wax or shave your hairy back, chest, arms and legs. Trim your armpits. **Hair Below the Belt**, you can trim or shave. Manscaping will show that you care about grooming, it'll make you look sexier, and it can increase sexual passion with your mate.

MIND YOUR MANNERS (Use social etiquette when out)

*There is something very sexy and attractive
about a man with good manners.*

*Y*our excellent physical appearance and your good manners will open doors, not just in your professional and social life, but in your personal life, as well. Say, "please" and "thank you," when it is fitting. Open the doors for her. When you open a car door for her help her in and then making sure that she is all in, close the door. At the dinner table, pull the chair out for her to sit, and then push the chair in. If she gets up from the table stand up to help with her chair (if possible). Know your dinning etiquette well and use it. Be familiar with the choice of wine or champagne. When entertaining, be a gracious host conscious of the right etiquette and amenities. Have good posture whether sitting or walking (this will also help to keep your body looking young). It is also important for you to increase your verbal and non-verbal communication skills.

Chivalry is alive and well!

AT HOME

*W*ear sexy or attractive loungewear home-line for men; try to look your best even at home. Help her to keep the house clean, neat, and smelling good. Work on having a peaceful atmosphere (the way you keep your home is a reflection of your spirit and soul).

Benilda Nya

You Can Only Eat An Elephant One Bite At A Time.

Sunday

Whoever watches the wind will not plant; whoever looks at the clouds will not reap. Ecclesiastes 11: 4

Monday

Express your love for her in her favorite cartoon by photocopying it and rewriting in the original captions.

Tuesday

Accept her imperfections, and just concentrate on her strengths.

Wednesday

Your happiness does not depend on her, but it is for you to create.

Thursday

Ask her if there is anything that she needs your help with to achieve her goals.

Friday

Never take for granted or get dispassionate about her giving you gifts and showing her love and appreciation to you.

Saturday

Ride a bicycle built for two.

NOTES:

Daily Coaching—Week 29

Be Your Best

*E*ven your yard (front and back) or balcony reflects on your personality. Your home is your castle, so make it a beautiful and pleasant place to live in. If you really want to impress her, you can also practice etiquette (social and dining) at home once in a while. If your wife works outside the home, you both can take turns to prepare the food the night before so that who ever gets home first can start to cook dinner.

COMMUNITY LIAISON

*G*et involved in your community: vote, volunteer with your wife to help with community projects (but do not over do it and neglect your home). Help those in need, feed the hungry, and clothe the naked, help the fatherless and widows. Be a good neighbor. Become a mentor. Join a good house of worship; church/synagogue.

HAVE A PLEASING PERSONALITY

*I*t is a pleasure to be around nice people. Be a man of excellence. Be prudent, use discernment and have integrity. Be a man of strength and dignity. When you speak, let your words be wise. Add to that self-control and organization, and let that be your guide to success. Be energetic and have a positive outlook about yourself, your marriage, your family, life and people; it will attract a lot of good things to you.

FINANCIALLY SAVVY

*C*heap things are never good, so watch for bargains to make your purchases. Plan the budget with your wife and stick to it. Use those coupons, and get those rebates. Shop smart. Learn to manage your money by diligently tracking your spending. Make informed financial decisions.

SELF HELP

*R*echarge and refuel yourself. Replenish your spirit, soul and body. Get yourself a mentor or two. Learn to discern who is a friend and who is an acquaintance, or who is a work buddy or just a fellow employee. Use wisdom in what you say and how much you say and to whom. Choose to be happy, and to be grateful.

Benilda Nya

What You Do Daily Will Determine Your Future.

Sunday

Lazy hands make a man poor, but diligent hands brings wealth. Proverbs 10: 4

Monday

Take a walk hand in hand or go for a drive after dinner & tell your wife that you'd rather be with her right there than any other place in the world. (Feel it.)

Tuesday

Make breakfast and make up the bed.

Wednesday

WARNING: use if appropriate for both of you. *Make love in a different place: the backyard, balcony, at the beach, at the park, in the car, on your boat/yacht. Please make sure that you have privacy, and do this only if appropriate for both of you.*

Thursday

Preparation is the key to handling the opportunities and obstacles along the way.

Friday

Have a candle light dinner in the backyard or balcony.

Saturday

Read to one another in bed.

NOTES/COMMENTS/JOURNAL: (Keep a record of what worked, changes made or new ideas.)

Daily Coaching – Week 30

There's always a reason to Celebrate!

❤ *H*ow do you feel when you celebrate? Do you get happy and full of enthusiasm? Then you should copy this euphoric feeling as often as possible.

❤ *T*hrow a party to celebrate yourself, your wife, your marriage, your loved ones or just to simply rejoice about life itself. Celebrate this beautiful planet that God created for you to get pleasure from, because He wants you to live your life with significance and determination.

Benilda Nya

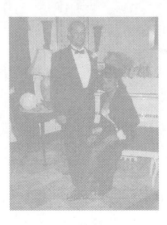

(Place a picture here of you and your spouse at a party.)

With Prosperity Comes The Responsibility Of Purpose.

Sunday

The Lord will send a blessing on your barns and on everything you put your hand to. The Lord your God will bless you in the land He is giving you. Deuteronomy 28: 8

Monday

Buy her a couple of gifts and hide them in places where she can find them throughout the week.

Tuesday

Make breakfast.
After dinner, do some cheek-to-cheek dancing by candlelight.

Wednesday

Dedicate a song to her on her favorite radio station (make sure she's listening).

Thursday

Get good at forgiving, because people will always disappoint you.

Friday

Help her to set the dinner table, candles and all.

Saturday

Give a beach party with your wife for your friends and relatives.

NOTES:

Daily Coaching – Week 31

*E*ncourage her to share her sexual fantasies with you and whenever possible, surprise her by taking the lead and making it happen. What ever it might be, do not make her feel weird or silly and just play with the ones that you are comfortable with and/or arouse you.

Benilda Nya

Don't Just Exist ... Live Everyday With Purpose And Reach Your Potential.

Sunday

Tickle her, and then kiss her all over.

... then nothing they plan to do will be impossible for them. Genesis 11: 6

Monday

Bring home her favorite dessert. (If you have children bring them their favorite, also.)

Tuesday

Take time out for fun and games.

Wednesday

Go for a walk with arms around each other, and tell her that she's an amazing woman.

Thursday

Be friendly and fun to be with.

Friday

Stop her in the middle of a conversation, look at her and tell her how gorgeous she is.

Saturday

Go out for breakfast. Afterwards go to the park and go boating and/or horseback riding. If it is possible, make out with her on the boat or a private spot somewhere in the park.

NOTES/COMMENTS/JOURNAL: (Keep a record of what worked, changes made or new ideas.)

Daily Coaching – Week 32

Honor Her

Tell her how valuable she is to you.

....

Love her by sacrificing for her.

....

Work out the disagreements.

....

Make her your top priority.

....

Be willing to do for her.

....

Be committed to her.

....

Be her best friend.

Benilda Nya

When You Give To Help Those In Need, You Open The Doors For Wonderful Things To Come To You.

Sunday

A generous man will prosper; he who refreshes others will himself be refreshed. Proverbs 11: 25

Monday

Float together in the pool, or go for a night swim.

Tuesday

Do not get bored with the daily practice of fundamentals.

Wednesday

Whenever she takes you out on a date, away for the weekend or does something extraordinary, send her a gift (to her job or home) with a thank you card.

Thursday

Gladly do what she asks you to do.

Friday

Call her during the day and ask her out on a date.

Saturday

Wine and dine, reminisce together; create some new memories.

NOTES:

Daily Coaching – Week 33

$\mathcal{L}$ove Notes

- Make a flyer; advertising the event that you want to take place: "The Love Doctor will be in town on _____, all those interested in the Love seminar, please join him at _____. Come ready for Love in all the right places."
- If you want to make her a delicious dinner: "Chef of Love" will be cooking up some pleasurable taste's on ____. See-through attire is a must. Dessert will be "ON" the chef.
- Write a poem on beautiful parchment paper, scroll it, tie with a ribbon, spray it lightly with your signature cologne and have it hand-delivered to her.
- Write her a thank you note (for a great time or for something special she did for you).
- Send her a formal invite with an RSVP the next time you want to give her an extraordinary surprise.
- If you are traveling, send her a postcard every day that you are away.
- Audio/video tape a sexy, love message.
- Send her the appropriate colored roses or flowers with the coordinating love note. For example: send her Pink and White roses with a note that says, "I LOVE YOU STILL AND ALWAYS WILL." Or Yellow and Orange roses with an invitation to get away for a passionate weekend rendezvous with you.
- Write her a love note in the personal section of your city's newspaper. Find your note and circle it with a heart then place it where she can see it.
- Make her her own personal "sexy" 5x7 or 8x10 calendar of yourself. Take lots of pictures in twelve different outfits and looks in a variety of poses: sexy, erotic, sweet (make sure your eyes talk to her). You can make this a "photo shoot date" and take pictures of each other to create your personal calendars together. Great foreplay!

Search in the Bible for "The Song of Solomon" (second book after Proverbs); it is full of sexy and beautiful poems that you can use. You can also go to the Library or bookstore and find books that can help you write poems and love letters.

Benilda Nya

Get Wisdom.

Sunday

Blessed is the man who finds wisdom, and the man who gains understanding. Proverbs 3: 13

Monday

Keep her madly in love.

Tuesday

Give her a compliment daily. Be specific.

Wednesday

Ask her how her day was. Put her to bed and give her a massage.

Thursday

With practice, you can make yourself happier.

Friday

Enrich your relationship; tell her "I love you."

Saturday

Have a captivating attitude with her.

NOTES/COMMENTS/JOURNAL: (Keep a record of what worked, changes made or new ideas.)

Daily Coaching – Week 34

Build and/or Decorate Your House
With Romance in Mind

- **Overall Design:** large windows, arched doorways, and high ceilings. Split levels, columns, sky lights, atriums and spacious rooms. Beautiful doors and hardware. Water fountain.
- **Sunken Living room:** columns, arched doorways, tray ceiling, wall water fall/fountain. Silk or chiffon/sheer drapes. Shaggy rug, wood, marble or glass tile flooring with a shaggy area rug.
- **Family room:** fireplace, silk/chiffon/velvet drapes.
- **Game Room/area:** velvet drapes, pool table, card/board games, ping-pong or hockey table and video games.
- **Media Room:** surround sound screen T.V. Fluffy oversized "L" or "U" shaped leather (or other soft fabric) sofa, oversized reclining chairs and a center table.
- **Library:** leather wing chairs and sofa, floor-to-ceiling built in mahogany bookshelves with a ladder to reach upper shelves, and a computer station.
- **Master Bedroom:** fireplace, top of the line mattress and four poster/canopy bed, decorative iron or upholstered headboard with fabric draping from the ceiling to the floor. Chandelier above the bed, if possible, or wall lighting sconces for soft lighting; scented candles. A vase with fresh roses on the nightstand. Crisp or silky linen (with high tread count), and if there is room for a sitting area, create a sensual setting with extra large decorative pillows, a furry floor rug and a low upholstered coffee table. And a stereo to play some of that romantic music you have.
- **Master Bathroom:** shower built for two with multiple showerheads and a built-in seat. Roman/Jacuzzi tub built for two with air jets and heater. A chandelier, curtains and aromatic candles are a must.
- **Dining Room:** with beautiful furniture, columns; chandelier, and trim the windows with silk or chiffon drapes.
- **Your Balcony:** can also be a nest for "romance" depending on where and how it is facing. You can put plants, torches, a hammock, white outdoor curtains, patio furniture or add a café table so that you may enjoy eating outside.

Benilda Nya

How Are You Handling The Difficult Things In Life?
Your Children Are Watching and Learning.

Sunday

Children's children are a crown to the aged, and parents are the pride of their children. Proverbs 17: 6

Monday

See the "challenge" in a trial not the burden.

Tuesday

Be charming with her. Nurture her. Sweet-talk her.

Wednesday

Improve your sex appeal.

Thursday

Be proud of your body.

Friday

If she gets home after you, greet her at the door with a big hug and kiss.

Saturday

Have an emotional interaction… share deep feelings.

NOTES:

Daily Coaching – Week 35

- **Backyard:** landscape with security and privacy in mind. You'll need it to be able to enjoy "romantic" moments in the swimming pool or hot tub. If your pool or hot tub areas do not have a waterfall design, then buy or make your own. You can also build or buy a pond with a waterfall design and fill it with water plants and gold fish. Create a beautiful and romantic area for eating outdoors. Build a cabana, loggia, sitting and/or lounging area with a theme: Moroccan, Roman, Spanish, Jungle look, etc. Install a beautiful birdbath and plant flowers that will attract butterflies and humming birds. If possible, have an outdoor sound system (be considerate of your neighbors, keep the volume low to moderate).
- **Party Room/Area:** design a sound proof room where you can build a small stage with stage lighting. Maybe add a sliding pole, curtains and a nice backdrop. Have a beverage area/bar with countertop and stools and a dance floor. For sitting, use low, upholstered platforms topped with extra big decorative pillows. Trim the walls with mirrors, the windows with ceiling to floor curtains, low center tables and soft lighting. The sound system should be well equipped with the best music of every category that you both enjoy, especially romantic music. I'm sure you, your wife and children (if any) can use that stage for private or family performances. (If you can't have a "party room," then designate a corner or area in the living room or family room where you can build a small platform with spotlights.)
- **In your car:** keep a "love basket" equipped with a towel, blanket, etcetera. Whether in the car, on the beach, at the park or your favorite scenic view, you can be prepared for those planned or spontaneous "romantic" encounters with your wife.
- **If you rent:** you can still decorate your place to be really romantic by the size and shape of your furniture and the fabrics that you choose. Have floor-to-ceiling drapes, a framed mirror in the dining room, candles wall sconces/stands, candles in the bathroom, and bedroom. Accent with throw rugs, decorative pillows, fresh flowers and your favorite scents. A great sound system is a must for your favorite music (be considerate of your neighbors, keep the volume low to moderate).

A clean and well-organized home is always a plus when it comes to enriching the "romantic" atmosphere in your home. The house should always have fresh flowers and in-door plants, candles, maybe even a water fountain and it should smell great.

Benilda Nya

Wisdom Has Great Benefits.

Sunday

Wisdom will prolong your life many years and bring you prosperity. The wise inherit honor. Proverbs 3: 2, 35

Monday

Clean up the kitchen after dinner.

Tuesday

Wake her up with your sweet kisses.

Wednesday

Make it a "spa date;" make two appointments for Saturday at her favorite spa; you both deserve some serious pampering. (Let her know that you are taking her on a "spa date.")

Thursday

After dinner, call her over to the couch and cuddle with her while watching TV.

Friday

When she takes you out on a date, look good, smell good be on your best behavior and have fun.

Saturday

Enjoy your well-deserved pampering.

NOTES/COMMENTS/JOURNAL: (Keep a record of what worked, changes made or new ideas.)

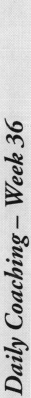

Daily Coaching – Week 36

ℐut on your Marriage Armor

(So that you can stand against the schemes that lead to betrayal & divorce.)

❤ **Belt of Truth:** you love your mate that is why you chose her. Ask her (with the right attitude, at a time of intimacy) for what you need that she might not be giving you, instead of trying to find it in someone or something else. Spend quality time together with your mate. Nurture your relationship with her; do not get wrapped up into working so hard to make ends meet or being an overachiever that you leave no room for the family. If you don't nurture your relationship, you and your family will suffer the consequences, so please find a good balance.

❤ **Breastplate:** safeguard against spending time with the wrong people: a man that is not interested in the sanctity of marriage or that might disrespect your wife or children, or a woman with her own agenda. Protect yourself at work too; avoid spending private time with other women, or with a woman that you might find interesting or attractive. In addition, you must watch what you talk about with other women; it should not be anything that is intimate or sexual because these subjects have been known to start a sexual relationship, even between people who where not looking to go astray or found each other interesting or attractive. That is another reason why being intimate with your mate is imperative for a healthy relationship.

❤ **Feet built-in:** be ready to immediately walk away from the circumstances that will be detrimental for your marriage, your personal and professional life. Do not look for the wrong things to fill any voids in your marriage.

Benilda Nya

Visualize And Plan Your Perfect Week.

Sunday

The plans of the diligent lead to profit… Proverbs 21: 5

Monday

Before she goes to bed, tell her and show her that you value her. Cuddle and kiss her, make her some tea.

Tuesday

Call her before you get home and ask her what she would like for dessert.

Wednesday

Have peace and faith in the midst of trials.

Thursday

Show her and tell her how much you admire her.

Friday

Enhance your relationship; tell her "I am so in love with you."

Saturday

Empower yourself with courage to do the things that you know you must do, even though you may not want to do them.

NOTES:

Daily Coaching – Week 37

Put on your Marriage Armor

(So that you can stand against the schemes that lead to betrayal & divorce.)

❤ **Shield:** have faith in God, yourself and in your mate for a successful relationship. This faith will put out those flaming arrows that will attack you and try to sabotage your integrity, your present and your future. Pray for your marriage and family daily.

❤ **Helmet:** protect your eyes; control your mind and your thoughts. What you think about and visualize is what will happen. (If you see that the grass looks greener on the other side, it is only because somebody was willing to nurture, fertilize, water and pull out the weeds, or it's a facade.)

❤ **Sword:** intimacy, sexual and verbal communication. Focus on the attention needed to fulfill one another. Your marriage is not just a fifty/fifty effort, but it is for both of you to give a hundred percent, even two-hundred percent or more.

BREATHE In Deeply, Exhale Slowly, And THINK Before You Speak.

Sunday

A gentle answer turns away wrath, but a harsh word stirs up anger. Proverbs 15: 1

Monday

Take her to the movies. Kiss her and caress her while watching the movie.

Tuesday

Renew your mind (the way you perceive things).

Wednesday

Keep the home fire burning hot, hotter and hottest!

Thursday

Smile at her, look at her with passion.

Friday

Praise her for not being a high maintenance woman.

Saturday

Make plans to take a vacation at a very romantic place.

Look at and caress her lips, tell her that her lips are "so soft" then kiss her.

NOTES/COMMENTS/JOURNAL: (Keep a record of what worked, changes made or new ideas.)

Daily Coaching – Week 38

When she gets home tired from work...

💜 **S**urprise her with a nice, hot bath with lavender oil and a long, back or full body massage (15-30 minutes).

💜 **P**amper her with a luxurious, hot foot soak with Epsom salt and lavender oil, followed by a foot massage; especially if she worked on her feet all day.

💜 **T**reat her to a gentle neck, shoulders and head massage and her favorite drink (if her job drains her because of all the thinking she has to do).

💜 **B**eing a homemaker more than qualifies her for the above treats, also.

💜 **G**ive her the royal treatment when she comes back from a business trip: pick her up in a limo (find out ahead of time what she would like to eat, and have it ready for her to eat along with her favorite wine/champagne or beverage in the limo). Eat and drink on the drive home (make sure that the driver takes his time and maybe even take the scenic view drive).

Benilda Nya

Check And Double Check Your Motives.

All a man's ways seem innocent to him, but motives are weighed by the Lord. Proverbs 16: 2

Believe in yourself.

Wake her up by kissing her and saying, "I Love You."

Work and play at being romantic.

Clean up the kitchen after dinner; make her her favorite beverage.

Have a good and vast selection of games to play. You can also buy a karaoke machine and sing to each other.

Serenade her: hire a band/singer for a couple of hours to play/sing before, during and after dinner.
(Dress sexy and look your best, put on her favorite cologne and use your social and dinner etiquette.)

If you play the piano, keyboard, harp, violin, flute, saxophone or guitar, play for her. If you sing, then sing a song to her.

NOTES:

Daily Coaching — Week 39

*H*er Mighty Fortress

Her Protector

❤ **F**rom the landscaping and the lighting outside of the house to the doors and windows and the inside of the house, make sure that your home is well-protected against intruders. Have an alarm that can function even if the phone lines are cut.

❤ **W**hen at home, the windows and doors should have a chime to let you know if they are opened.

❤ **I**f you are going out of town and she is staying home, make sure that all safety devices are working; tell trusted friends or family to check on her.

❤ **C**reate a safety room in the house, or a way out in case of fire or danger.

❤ **Y**ou can call her when you arrive at your destination, and also call her a couple of times during the day and before she goes to bed; remind her to turn on the house alarm.

Benilda Nya

Sow Seeds Of Kindness... Be Kind To Yourself And Others.

Sunday

A kind man benefits himself, but a cruel man brings trouble on himself. Proverbs 11: 17

Monday

Respect yourself, so that others can also respect you.

Tuesday

Tickle her, kiss her all over and tell her how beautiful she is.

Wednesday

Flirt with her while talking.

Thursday

Romantic love is exclusive for your lifetime commitment.

Friday

Have an inspiring conversation with her, and create excitement with your tone of voice.

Saturday

Join her in a nice and hot aromatherapy bubble bath and talk about your dreams and goals. (When you are done, help her to clean up the bathtub.)

NOTES/COMMENTS/JOURNAL: (Keep a record of what worked, changes made or new ideas.)

Daily Coaching – Week 40

A Safe Haven

❤ **T**he car should have an alarm and a prompt recovery device.

❤ **S**he should carry some type of protection in her purse.

❤ **T**ake some form of personal protection class; you can make it a family time event.

❤ **M**ake your home a "green" home. Buy organic/natural as much as possible: foods, personal hygiene products, hair and skin care products, cosmetics, household cleaners, bedding, furnishings and accessories. Improve the quality of your water by using a filtration system, and an air purifying system will give you and your family better air to breath. You can also buy indoor plants that help clean the air inside your home. When painting and/or remodeling the house use organic/non-toxic paints and supplies. You can also improve the air inside your car with an Auto Ionizer.

Benilda Nya

To Increase Your Chances For An Excellent And Healthy Life; Help Each Other To Fulfill Your Hopes And Dreams.

Sunday

Go out for brunch and afterwards take her ice-skating; hold hands while skating.

Hope deferred (postponed/delayed) makes the heart sick, but a longing fulfilled is a tree of life. Proverbs 13: 12

Monday

Improve your problem solving skills.

Tuesday

Bring home her favorite cake or pie for dessert; serve and/or feed it to her after dinner.

Wednesday

Have a movie night at home: buy or make hers and your favorite movie snacks, cover yourselves with a blanket and cuddle as you watch the movie.

Thursday

Sneak up behind her, fondle her and kiss her neck.

Friday

Life is not perfect, people are not perfect, relationships are not perfect, so do not expect perfection. People and circumstances will disappoint you, so just learn from the mistakes and try to see the good that can come from the experience; always do your best to look for the decent qualities in people.

Saturday

Enjoy your date with her when she takes you out.

Her Refuge

- ❤ **If** she drives, make sure that the car is in good shape and well-maintained. Go fill it up for her, and have it washed. Teach her how to check the oils, the battery and how to change a flat (make sure that all the tools and the spare tire are there and in proper shape).

- ❤ **These** days a cell phone is no longer a luxury, but a necessity. Make sure you both have one and, if the children are old enough, they too, should have one. You can also invest in a satellite phone just incase you need one.

- ❤ **Does** she have a bicycle? Maintain it for her, but also teach her how to take care of it.

Go ahead and take pleasure in protecting her and in being her "Knight in Shining Armor" because, this type of caring and nurturing will show her how much you love and value her. That will also increase her desire to please you, and it could intensify her passion for sexual romance!

Benilda Nya

With The Proper Balance, Work Hard For Your Marriage And Your Career.

Sunday

If she wants to serve breakfast in bed, indulge yourselves.

All hard work brings a profit... Proverbs 14: 23

Monday

Before going to sleep, caress her face; look at her and tell her that she's got you hypnotized.

Tuesday

Be aware of what she needs and give it to her, without her having to ask.

Wednesday

Play out one of her sexual fantasies (do it right).

Thursday

Celebrate your accomplishments.

Friday

Continue to polish your plans; strive for excellence.

Saturday

Touch her and look at her when you speak to her.

If she is going away on a business trip, make some real good, long love to her the night before, or if possible, in the morning of the day that she is leaving. Write her a love note; tell her how much you'll miss her and give her your well wishes, spray it with your signature fragrance then put it in a plastic sandwich bag. Sneak into her packed bag and place the note where she can see it when she opens the bag. Or, you could have an arrangement of flowers with a love note, delivered to her wherever she is going to stay.

NOTES/COMMENTS/JOURNAL: (Keep a record of what worked, changes made or new ideas.)

Daily Coaching — Week 42

Forever Pleasing Her
10 Commandments

1. Cultivate your marriage with words: "I'm in love with you." "Thank you." "Please." How can I help? "I appreciate you." "I was wrong." "I'm sorry." "I forgive you." "I can't imagine my life without you." "You are so beautiful." "I love it when you _____." etc.

2. Communicate / Connect / Listen: be honest about your feelings, share your thoughts and dreams/goals, help her to understand you. Listen to her, encourage and understand her. Be patient; talk about decisions together, it takes time to develop a meaningful communication. Look at conflicts as the doorway to better intimacy and wisdom, so deal with them openly and directly.

3. Be physical and passionate: hug, kiss, caress & flirt. Celebrate and praise her, contribute in all duties, aim to please her, look your best.

4. Lead by your actions: set a good example, plant what you want to harvest, if you want more and lasting success – pray daily with your wife/family.

5. Give your mate the freedom to think for herself: her originality and intelligence will increase your own. Relax, do not require for your mate and children to act exactly like you and do things the way that you do.

6. There is no place for: unresolved anger, manipulation and harsh criticism.

7. Be fun to live with.

8. Live beyond the blame game.

9. Make deposits: have a positive attitude, lend an ear, a helping hand, non-sexual romance, thoughtfulness, kindness. **Not withdrawals:** Being unappreciative, selfish, negative words and attitude, unkind or unreliable.

10. As much as possible, position your spouse to receive the best first: by doing that you will create a marriage that surpasses all wedding-day dreams, where love not only lasts, but it grows constantly. The honeymoon is on a continual basis.

Benilda Nya

What Is Your Face Saying About You?

Sunday

A happy heart makes the face cheerful, but heartache crushes the spirit.
Proverbs 15: 13

Monday

Handle money the right way.

Tuesday

When possible, look into her eyes while she talks to you.

Wednesday

Enjoy her naughtiness.

Thursday

Smile and be happy; feel like the amazing hot man that you are.

Friday

Be interested in what she likes to do: hobbies, work, sports, etc.

Saturday

Be open and transparent with each other.

Honor your love for her: give her a kiss if you are the one who is right in a discussion or disagreement.

NOTES:

Daily Coaching – Week 43

The Ordinary VS The Extraordinary Life

The Ordinary Life (The Basics)

Work, pay the rent/mortgage, pay the bills, car payment(s), groceries, sex once a week. Helping with the house chores, helping with the children, making sure that things around the house are in good shape (that things are not falling apart or breaking).

The Expected Essentials

Home furnishings, replenishing clothes and shoes. Sending her to the beauty salon once or twice a month, and you going to the barber once or twice a month. Leisure: movies/dinner etc. (once or twice a month). The expected gifts: something for: her Birthday, Anniversary, Valentine's Day, Mother's Day, Christmas, (a common show of affection).

The "basics" are for a functioning life and home. The "expected" Essentials, are the things that you as the man of the house and the provider should be able to supply in addition to the basics. Whether she works at home as a homemaker or is a career woman, these are your basic and expected requirements for the marriage covenant. (Be careful with these, for they can be a very boring and monotonous way to live.)

The Extraordinary Life

- **Work**: whether you work at home, have your own business or work for somebody else, you are happy to do what you do and you do it with excellence and integrity.
- **Bills/Finances:** pay the rent/mortgage, and Car payment(s) before the due date. Pay the full amount you spent on your credit cards on the due date, or pay double or more of the minimum payment due. Pay two or more car and mortgage payments whenever possible.

Benilda Nya

"Every Day You Are On The Way." Where Are You Going?

Sunday

A greedy man brings trouble to his family, but he who hates bribes will live. Proverbs 15: 27

Monday

Never get tired of going out of your way to please and excite her.

Tuesday

Talk sexy and drive her wild.

Wednesday

Do not crowd her; give her space.

Thursday

Use common sense.

Friday

Take your creativity to the next level.

Saturday

Take her to the park for a carriage ride.

NOTES/COMMENTS/JOURNAL: (Keep a record of what worked, changes made or new ideas.)

Daily Coaching – Week 44

The Extraordinary Life

- **Groceries:** when you go grocery-shopping buy the best and the healthiest foods. Buy her her favorite foods to eat, as well as her favorite brands of toiletries and cleaning items. If you have children, buy their favorites too.
- **Intimacy:** living a life of *non-sexual* romance, and pleasurable *sexual* romance (sex in a variety of places and ways), more than once a week. Wear nice loungewear around the house every day to be her "eye candy." Treat her like royalty.
- **Help with the house chores:** keep the house clean (clean the way she likes it). Pick-up and cleanup (especially after yourself). With her approval, you can hire a maid once a week or month to do these house chores.
- **Help with the children:** get the children ready for bed and school, help them with their homework. Take them to and from sport activities. Read to them in bed and pray with them.
- **Make sure that things around the house are in good shape:** with her approval hire a trusted handyman to fix things around the house to help you.
- **The laundry:** when washing and drying the clothes, you could iron them or fold them nicely and put them away in the correct closets and drawers. With her approval you can also send the laundry to be washed. Take to the cleaners the clothes that need it. If you want to be considered for that promotion and increase your financial status, your clothes should always look the part.
- **Home furnishings:** should never be worn out or broken. Replace things around the house before they get old and ugly. Keep a beautifully furnished home; you can do this even on a tight budget. Ask your wife about things that need replacing or fixing, give her money to buy something new for the house (without her having to ask).

Get Rid Of Your Negative Emotions.

Sunday

Each heart knows its own bitterness, and no one else can share its joy.
Proverbs 14: 10

Monday

On a cold winter night, make some hot chocolate with whipped cream for the both of you.

Tuesday

When she wants to get it on, give her a mind-boggling, body quivering orgasm.

Wednesday

Use your brain properly: envision yourself acting and responding to stressful or negative situations and people the proper way. By doing this, you will learn to change your mind.

Thursday

Avoid negative criticism; be understanding, loving and sincere.

Friday

Have dinner and dessert in bed, surrounded by candlelight, and talk about your first date.

Saturday

Be happy to experience life together.

Send her a hand-delivered, hand-written invitation on fancy parchment paper wrapped in ribbon. Invite her to get away with you in a mountain cabin or ski lodge.

NOTES:

Daily Coaching – Week 45

The Extraordinary Life

- **Replenishing clothes and shoes:** take your wife, your kids (if you have kids) and yourself shopping for new clothes and shoes other than when needed.
- **Going to the beauty salon/barber:** if the budget does not stretch for regular visits to the salon and barber, then learn how to maintain the look until the next visit. If your budget permits send her to the salon every week.
- **Take her out to eat:** make it a four-or five-star restaurant, (even if it's on a quarterly basis), especially on her birthday, your wedding anniversary and Valentine's Day.
- **Give her the flower of the month bouquet/basket every month.**
- **Surprise her:** give her jewelry just because you know it will look great on her, or because you know she will love it, or just because she's worth it.

Extraordinary means that you will go the extra mile to please your spouse just because you enjoy making her happy and you delight in showing your love, appreciation and respect for her. You should be devoted to and concerned about the things that are important to her. Whenever possible, put a especial touch on what you do for her. When your aim is to please her, that's when you'll know that you are giving her an extraordinary and excellent marriage.

Benilda Nya

Be Careful With What You Allow To Enter You.

Sunday

Hold on to instruction, do not let it go; guard it well, for it is your life. Proverbs 4: 13

Monday

Rub her feet, head or back before going to sleep.

Tuesday

Keep on getting better; keep improving yourself and your techniques.

Wednesday

Bake some cookies, warm up some milk and take it to bed for both of you. (Include the kids if any.)

Thursday

You can't change each other, but if you give and take, and appreciate her, your lives will go a lot smoother.

Friday

Build her up in accordance with her need.

Saturday

Before you go to sleep: gaze into her eyes, caress her face, kiss her and tell her that you are totally wild about her.

NOTES/COMMENTS/JOURNAL: (Keep a record of what worked, changes made or new ideas.)

Daily Coaching – Week 46

Husbands...

Give honor to your wife. Treat her with understanding and be considerate as you live together, with an intelligent recognition (of the marriage relation). She might be (physically) weaker than you are, but she is your equal partner in God's gift of life. If you don't treat her as you should, your prayers will not be heard.

Proverb

RESPECT Your Money.

Sunday

Dishonest money dwindles away, but he who gathers money little by little makes it grow. Proverbs 13: 11

Monday

Accompany each other to doctor/dentist appointments.

Tuesday

On a cold morning or night, warm up her terry cloth slippers, robe and her towel; hand them to her after her shower.

Wednesday

Do something different, new, exciting or different in bed tonight.

Thursday

When she talks about the visions you share, tell her how capable and talented she is.

Friday

Add some sizzle to your weekend; go spend the night in her favorite hotel (in the honeymoon suite). Get dressed up for bed like you did for your honeymoon and stir up the flames of lust.

Saturday

Do the little things, they count too.

Pick a night next week when you can sit down with your wife (and older children, if any). Take pen and paper, and design the way that you want your new year to be. Write down your wants, needs, dreams, goals and the steps that need to be taken to accomplish these dreams and goals. Decide to create the right attitude by making the choices that will take you there.

Daily Coaching – Week 47

*Y*ou and your spouse should work on creating an excellent atmosphere in your home, so that your home is one of the best and safest places; a lifeline that you can cling to to have peace and joy, a place where you are able to de-stress and get away from the not so great things and people in your day. Your home is your castle, your hiding place and sanctuary. It should be a place for rejuvenation; make your home your spa away from the spa. Let yourself be these things for your wife and children, as well.

*T*ake time out every day to de-brief, so that you can prevent burnout. *Choose* to encourage yourself for improving the quality of your marriage and thus, refining the quality of your life.

*L*ife is about choices. So choose to love yourself and others; choose to be happy and to have integrity; choose peace and excellence. These things will only help you to reach your goals and to live your dreams.

Benilda Nya

Pursue Wisdom.

Sunday

The wisdom of the prudent is to give thought to their ways… Proverbs 14: 8

Monday

On a cold night, warm up the bed with an electric blanket, then carry her to bed and tuck her in.

Tuesday

Tell her, "I love you" in French… "Je T'adore."(See page 218 for saying "I love you" in other languages)

Wednesday

Make the morning coffee/tea, cut some fresh fruit and serve her and yourself.

Thursday

Persist in the pursuit of a "blissful" marriage; it is achievable.

Friday

Learn about your spouse's character (nature, disposition, tendencies).

Saturday

What is it about her that you find sexy? Tell her next time you make love to her.

NOTES/COMMENTS/JOURNAL: (Keep a record of what worked, changes made or new ideas.)

Daily Coaching – Week 48

Now It's the Time!

*E*njoy where you are at while on the way to where you are going

....

*S*top to smell the roses

....

*B*e aware of all the beautiful things around you

....

*Y*ou have the power to make everyday an extraordinary day

Benilda Nya

Keep Moving Forward!

*C*heck your mental vision; make sure that it is not distorted

....

*S*top functioning in your dysfunction

....

*Y*our past does not have to determine your future

....

*T*alk about yourself the way that you imagine
yourself to be/how youwant to be

....

*Y*ou yourself are a miracle and can make miracles happen; so never
stop hoping, believing, praying and giving and doing your best

Benilda Nya

Weekly Coaching

For the next four weeks, I want you to create the daily Non-Sexual and Sexual Romance ideas that your mate will love for you to carry out. I am sure that you will do an excellent job and enjoy doing it.

Sow Seeds Of Kindness... Be Kind To Yourself And Others.

Sunday

A kind man benefits himself, but a cruel man brings trouble on himself.
Proverbs 11: 17

Monday

Tuesday

Wednesday

Thursday

Friday

Saturday

NOTES:

Daily Coaching – Week 49

Weekly Coaching - Week 50

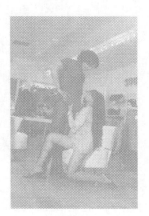

(Place a picture of both of you here.)

You Were Created To Succeed.

Sunday

A faithful man/woman will be richly blessed. Proverbs 28: 20

....

Monday

....

Tuesday

....

Wednesday

....

Thursday

....

Friday

....

Saturday

NOTES/COMMENTS/JOURNAL: (Keep a record of what worked, changes made or new ideas.)

Daily Coaching – Week 50

Communication in a relationship is crucial. Many couples fail to see the importance of their communication. When couples communicate effectively, they are able to understand each other better. Communication is a shared responsibility because it is a way of defining ourselves to our partner. It does not matter how old you are or how long you have been in your relationship, you still need to learn how to communicate your feelings and emotions to your partner. Your communication should be open and honest. It should not be used to create shame or guilt or ridiculing. An open and honest relationship with caring and sympathy is the key to a successful relationship.

An effective and warm listener can be a key to resolving conflicts when the relationship is failing. Communicating like "true friends" can enhance the time spent together. Couples need to find time alone, sit down together and discuss their concerns with each other more often than they do. When couples don't take the time to do this on a regular basis, other less effective ways of communicating such as gestures, tone of voice, anger, silence and rejection can become a normal part of your communication process. These means of communication are not only hurtful, but they also act as a barrier to building a strong relationship.

It is not a healthy manner of communicating to each other, but it sends a clear message to your partner that someone is not happy about something and chooses not to openly discuss the problem with his/her partner. It is sometimes a good idea to write a letter to your partner and try to be as open and honest as you can possibly be. Tell him/her how you feel. This is a good way of starting a conversation and to effectively convey a clear message to your partner that you do not want to continue feeling upset about something. The other partner's interpretation can be enhanced by asking questions and becoming an empathetic listener. It is sometimes difficult to have couples attentively listen without interrupting the other partner or becoming defensive. Keeping an open and non-judge mental attitude can help you build a more positive relationship. Maintaining open doors for more discussions can be another avenue to restart a conversation in the near future.

Continued

Become A Better You... Confront And Conquer Your Problems With A Positive Mental Attitude.

Sunday

...The desires of the diligent are fully satisfied. Proverbs 13: 4

Monday

Tuesday

Wednesday

Thursday

Friday

Saturday

NOTES/COMMENTS/JOURNAL: (Keep a record of what worked, changes made or new ideas.)

Daily Coaching – Week 51

We all need to be aware that our personal communication style may need to be enhanced. We may need to search ourselves first and make a personal inventory before we can understand our partner. Don't be afraid to research books and to educate yourself in how to become an effective listener and communicator. This will not only enhance your relationship with your partner, but it will enhance your relationship with your children and others in your life.

Article written by: Maritza Montano, PhD
    Licensed Mental Health Counselor
    Board Certified Counselor
    Diplomat of American Psychotherapist Association

If you would like more information regarding this topic, you can E-Mail Dr. Montano at: MLStres1@bellsouth.net

Motivate Yourself With A Positive Mental Attitude And You Will Also Motivate Your Mate And those Around You.

Sunday

A cheerful look brings joy to the heart, and good news gives health to the bones. Proverbs 11: 17

Monday

Tuesday

Wednesday

Thursday

Friday

Saturday

NOTES:

Daily Coaching – Week 52

Warning Against Adultery

My son, pay attention to my wisdom, listen well to my words of insight, that you may maintain discretion and your lips may preserve knowledge. For the lips of an adulteress drip honey, and her speech is smoother than oil; but in the end she is bitter as gall, sharp as a double-edged sword. Her feet go down to death; her steps lead straight to the grave. She gives no thought to the way of life; her paths are crooked, but she knows it not.

Now then, my sons, listen to me; do not turn aside from what I say. Keep to a path far from her, do not go near the door of her house, lest you give your best strength to others and your years to one who is cruel, lest strangers feast on your wealth and your toil enrich another man's house. At the end of your life you will groan, when your flesh and body are spent. You will say, "How I hated discipline! How my heart spurned correction! I would not obey my teachers or listen to my instructors. I have come to the brink of utter ruin in the midst of the whole assembly."

Drink water from your own cistern, running water from your own well. Should your springs overflow in the streets, your streams of water in the public squares? Let them be yours alone, never to be shared with strangers. May your fountain be blessed, and may you rejoice in the Wife of your youth. A loving doe, a graceful deer may her breasts satisfy you always, may you ever be captivated by her love. Why be captivated, my son, by an adulteress?

Why embrace the bosom of another man's wife?

For a man's ways are in full view of the Lord, and he examines all his paths. The evil deeds of a wicked man ensnare him; the cords of his sin hold him fast. He will die for lack of discipline, led astray by his own great folly.

Proverbs 5: 1–23 NIV

The Days of Heaven on Earth Can Be Yours

Form your own future with the words you speak. If things are not right within you, they will never be right around you. You also create your kids' future by what you speak into their lives. Love wisdom like a sweetheart; make wisdom a beloved member of your family.

You should get real about you. However, do not be too hard on yourself. Know that people are able to go to school to learn about everything except marriage and relationships, and few really teach on how to love and honor your spouse and family because this is something that is usually learned at home when growing up (if you were paying attention). You can also learn this when you are open and honest with yourself about what you need to learn about having a better marriage.

In coming into marriage, the two people should be whole: unique, with established standards, integrity and excellence not needy and in emotional, spiritual, physical, financial or moral disarray, hoping for a mate to complete them and provide all that is lacking. Marriage will show you who you truly are, because it will test your very last nerve. But it helps when you can celebrate your mate's uniqueness so that you can get from where you are to where you need to be. Marital bliss can be achieved; all you have to do is make a decision to make it so. It doesn't get any better than to live the rest of your life with someone who loves you and is committed to you in every way possible, someone who has your best interest at heart. Make it pleasurable, so that you and your mate can live the days of Heaven on Earth... as you Forever Please and Excite each other!

Benilda Nya

143

Part Three

Monthly Holidays and Event Coaching

January

Flower: Carnation, Snowdrop

Birthstone: Garnet–*constancy*

New Year's Day
Celebrated first in ancient Babylon about 4000 years ago, New Year's Day is the most ancient and universal of all holidays, and it often differs according to one's culture.

New Year's Day Traditions
New Year's Day is a day of parades, sporting events and new years resolutions. The Tournament of Roses Parade dates back to 1886, and it is followed by the Rose Bowl college football game.

To bring good luck
On the first day of the new year, eating anything in the shape of a circle is thought to bring good fortune by many cultures, because it represents "coming full circle." In most parts of the United States it is believed that eating legumes including black-eyed peas, as well as eating pig or cabbage is a sign of the expected prosperity for the new year.

For good luck, some cultures also believe in eating twelve grapes within the first few minutes of the new year, one for every month. In Israel, they eat apples dipped in honey on New Year's Day to bring a sweet year. The French, cheer the New Year with wine, champagne and a really special New Year's cake as a symbol of the sweet New Year that everyone wishes.

Another symbol that is connected with the New Year's celebration is that of a baby. This dates as far back as ancient Greece and Egypt as a universal symbol of rebirth, and it still finds its way into our modern celebrations as it represents the "baby New Year," in which all good things are possible.

"Auld Lang Syne"
Since the 1700s, the song, "Auld Lang Syne," is sung at the stroke of midnight in almost every English-speaking country in the world to bring in the new year. An old Scotch tune, "Auld Lang Syne" literally means "old long ago," "days gone by," "long long ago," or simply, "the good old days."

Meaningful Traditions and Things To Do On New Year's Day

New Year's Resolutions
The good old new years resolution tradition is said to have started with the Babylonians. Since so many of us make New Year's resolutions for a positive change, this is one of the most positive holidays that we can celebrate.

With this New Year comes the opportunity for a fresh and new start, as we say goodbye to the old year.

-Celebrating Tips
1. *New Year's Resolutions: Buy two 8X10 notebooks, one for each of you. Take time out with your spouse (include your children if they are old enough), talk about the things that you would like to accomplish for the new year as a couple as a family, and as individuals. Write down your personal and business goals, your "Mission" and "Vision" statements. Make your "Vision" board by cutting out pictures from magazines and newspapers with the things (clothes, car, home, toys) and situations/life style (your business, desired salary, net-worth, giving to your favorite foundation, etc.) that you want. Create a definite plan for carrying out your goals. Commit to reading your goals, mission and vision statements with passion twice daily. Once in the morning, soon after waking up and in the evening before going to sleep. Look at your vision board daily and be motivated, optimistic and grateful. Choose a quiet corner or area in your house, provide comfortable sitting and use it only to go over your mission and vision statements as well as to go over your affirmations.*

2. *Make a tradition out of releasing balloon wishes. Buy helium balloons in the colors that symbolize your desires for the new year. Purple means - power, royalty, luxury or elegance. Red - love, courage, desire, strength, determination, excitement or passion. Yellow - happiness, comfort, attention-grabbing, intellectual energy or optimism. Orange - stimulation, creativity, health or*

change. Green - well-being, nature, calm, growth, harmony or relaxation. Blue - peace, loyalty, honor, professionalism or trust. Gold - prosperity, wealth or wisdom. Silver - rich or glamour. Pink - sweet, playful or romance. Write each of your desires on paper, then attach each wish to the corresponding color balloon with a ribbon and release them into the sky within the first few minutes of the new year, say your affirmations for each goal and desire as they fly away. (Make a copy of the goals & desires you sent off and declare your affirmations daily and work your plan for achieving them.)

3. You can visit your family, friends and neighbors. Bring them some treats like cakes or cookies and your best wishes for the New Year.

4. Another great way to start the New Year is by helping those in need and by giving the gift of hope to those in need of inspiration.

5. Include your children if they are old enough to participate. Please take pictures!

6. End the first day of the year at home by... Making an excellent dinner with all the trimmings, and please use your finest dinner wear. Help her prepare dinner and cleanup afterwards.

Tu B'Shevat – Observed in January or February

Jewish Holidays happen on a different day every year because, the Jewish calendar coordinates with the rotation of the earth about its axis (a day), the revolution of the moon about the earth (a month), and the revolution of the earth about the sun (a year).

OTHER OBSERVANCES FOR THIS MONTH

National Blood Donor Month – If possible, donate blood and encourage others to do so.

- **National Thank You Month** – Say thank you more often.

- **National Eye Care Month** – Visit your eye care physician and have your eyes and those you love checked.

- **National Book Month**

- **Epiphany**

- Save the Eagles Day

- Amelia Earheart Day

- Ben Franklin's Birthday

- Martin Luther King Jr. Day

- Christa McAuliffe

- Chinese New Year

-Celebrating Tips

Celebrate the Chinese New Year. Join an oriental friend in their celebration or have a Chinese New Year dinner party (with some of the traditional foods), dress up, decorate the house, play Chinese music and end with some fire works outside the house and in the" bedroom."

Super Bowl Sunday
-Celebrating Tips

If she did something to help you enjoy Super Bowl Sunday, give her a big hug, a delicious kiss, thank her for understanding you, and tell her that she is your inspiration.

February

Flower: Violet, Primrose, Begonia

Birthstone: Amethyst--*sincerity*

Make this, a Valentine's Month, not just Day

-Celebrating Tips

1. *Give her a Valentine's gift every day for the month of February.*

2. *Give her daily, the color rose(s) or the number for the story of roses that express your feelings for her.*

Black History Month

Black History Month is a celebration to remember and learn more about the history and culture of black Americans.

National Freedom Day

Commemorates the signing of the 13th Amendment outlawing slavery on February 1, 1865 by President Lincoln.

Mardi Gras/Fat Tuesday

Mardi Gras, which in French translates to Fat Tuesday, is officially the day before Ash Wednesday. It occurs anytime between February 3rd and March 9th depending on when Easter is held that year.

"Let the Good Times Roll"

-Celebrating Tips

1. *Plan a trip to New Orleans for Mardi Gras.*
2. *Have a Mardi Gras style dinner party: music, food, beads, etc. (Plan it together with her.)*

Religious Holidays
-Celebrating Tips
1. *Celebrate your maker! A family that prays together and puts God first has a better chance of survival and happiness, so praise your spouse for their spiritual strength and/or leadership.*
2. *Statistics show that couples that do not pray together have a higher divorce rate than those that pray together.*

Valentine's Day

February 14th is the traditional day to express your love for each other. Celebrate this spirit of love by sending a valentine, giving candy or other gifts. There are two different legends of why we celebrate Valentine's Day... One legend started in Rome, when the Emperor, Claudius II, was involved in many bloody and unpopular campaigns. "Claudius the Cruel" as he was called, was having a difficult time getting soldiers to join his military leagues. He believed that the reason was that Roman men did not want to leave their loved ones. So, he cancelled all marriages and engagements in Rome.

The good Saint Valentine, who was a priest in Rome, in the year 269 A.D., together with his friend Saint Marius, defied Claudius and continued to perform marriages in secret. When Valentine's actions were discovered, he was sentenced to be beaten to death and have his head cut off.

While in prison, it is believed that Valentine fell in love with a young girl, who may have been his jailor's daughter, who visited him during his confinement. Before his death on the 14th day of February, it is alleged that he wrote her a letter, which he signed "From Your Valentine"

In 496 A.D., Pope Gelasius set aside February 14 to honor St. Valentine.

Happy Valentine's Day, Darling

- *Start by giving her a bouquet or arrangement of her favorite flowers or red roses the night before Valentine's Day.* *Plan this well in advance by calling the flower shop near your work or home to reserve the flowers. When you give them to her, let her know that: Valentine's Day is not long enough to show her how happy you are that she is your "Valentine."*

- *On Valentine's Day morning, wake her up with a kiss and say: "Happy Valentine's Day Darling(Baby)[Put name]," then give her a valentine's card* *and give her some jewelry. This jewelry could be something you know she wanted, or something to match or add to an existing piece she already has. Or you can start a tradition: give her a Ruby item/s (necklace and/or matching earrings or, bracelet and/or matching ring) every Valentine's Day until she has all the matching pieces. If she does not like Rubies, then make it her favorite stone.*

- *Give her her favorite stuffed animal in the biggest size you can get, along with a box of her favorite chocolates (or if she is on a special diet, fruits.)* *Have it delivered around mid-day to her work place or at home if she is home. Or you can deliver it yourself, and if possible, take her out to lunch or bring her some lunch.*

- *Surprise her by taking her out to dinner at a four- or five-star restaurant, or to her favorite place to eat. Go in style, rent a limousine.* *Give her a couple of days to get ready. Send her an invitation by mail, simple and elegant. Let her know how to dress: casual or dressy. If after dinner your plans are to take her to her favorite hotel for the night/weekend, let her know that she will need an overnight bag. Do not give away the surprise (the limousine and where you're taking her). Make all the appropriate reservations in advance. Make sure that you also look your best (wear the color & style that she loves to see you in). Be well groomed, put on her favorite Cologne.*

This is the perfect time to use excellent table and social manners. When she's finished getting dressed, tell her how beautiful she looks and smells. Throughout the evening: look at her, flirt with her, smile at her and caress her. Kiss her hand, lips, cheeks and shoulders (if they are bare). Tell her how beautiful she looks during dinner. If she looks sexy, tell her. Tell her what you love and admire about her and how you respect her. Tell her the ways that she has been a positive help and force in your life. The conversation should be positive and Romantic.

*- **Serenade her.** If you plan a romantic dinner at home for her, surprise her and hire a mariachi band, a local singer or group to serenade her during dinner.*

*- **Night of Passion.*** This is a great way to start or conclude Valentine's Day. If you ask her to meet you at the Hotel so that you can prepare the room/surprise, have her picked up by a limo service. (Make a list of all the things you'll need to bring.) If you are going there with her after dinner, make sure that you arrange all the details at the Hotel with concierge/guest services such as, rose petals on the bed, a tray full of the rose petals in the bathroom (so that you can put them in the bubble bath water after you draw it), the aromatic candles, fruit, finger food, champagne or wine. Bring the music with you.

Benilda Nya

End Valentine's Month by:

1. *Having a relaxing but sexy dinner with music and cheek-to-cheek dancing at home, with all the trimmings and etiquette. Plan it together with your spouse.*
2. *Write her a poem or letter about the great time you had for Valentine's Day, weekend or month, and send it to her by messenger delivery along with an arrangement of red Chrysanthemums (I Love you), or Gerberas (You are the Sunshine of My Life) or Lily-Of -The- Valley (You've Made My Life Complete). Spray your cologne on the letter.*

OTHER OBSERVANCES FOR THIS MONTH:

- **American Heart Month** – Keep a healthy heart.
- **National Dental Month** – A healthy mouth = Better health.
- **Chocolate Lovers Month**
- **National Bird Feeding Month**
- **Tu B'Shevat** – January or February
- **Purim** – February or March
- **Groundhog Day**
- **Ash Wednesday** – It occurs anytime between February 6th and March 9th, depending on when Easter is held that year.
- **Boy Scout Day**
- **Presidents' Day**

March

Flower: Daffodil, Jonquil

Birthstone: Aquamarine, Bloodstone–*courage*

Read Across America Day/Dr. Suess Birthday
-Celebrating Tips
Read poems to each other.

Palm Sunday
This is held on the Sunday before Easter Sunday, anytime between March and April, depending on when Easter is held that year.

St. Patrick's Day
-Celebrating Tips
Have a St. Patrick's Day theme dinner; don't forget the music.

First Day of Spring
-Celebrating Tips
After breakfast, clean the windows and help her do some Spring-cleaning. There is a delightful reward for being thoughtful.

Pesach (Passover) – March or April

Good Friday
It occurs anytime between March and April, depending on when Easter is held that year.

Easter Sunday
It occurs anytime between March 22nd and April 25th, on the first Sunday after the first full moon after March 20th.

ADDITIONAL OBSERVANCES FOR THIS MONTH

- **Purim** – February or March
- **National Nutrition Month** – Eat healthy and smart, and exercise
- **National Women's History Month** – Discover women's forgotten multicultural history and heritage.
- **Save Your Vision Week** – 1st week in March
- **Ash Wednesday** – February or March depending on when Easter is held that year.
- **Girl Scout Week 10-16**
- **National Poison Prevention Week** – 3rd week in March
- **Sea Turtles nesting period begins in Florida**
- **Daylight Savings Time** – Set clocks forward 1 hour.

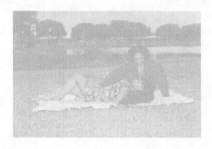

(Place a spring picture of the two of you here.)

Flower: Sweet Pea, Daisy

Birthstone: Diamond–*innocence*

April Fools'/All Fool's Day – 1st of April
-Celebrating Tips
You can pleasantly fool her by giving her April flowers (assorted colored Daisies) and diamond jewelry in a computer box.

April 15th Taxes Due
-Celebrating Tips
Be in a good mood; it will only get better.

Earth Day
-Celebrating Tips
1. *Go to your favorite beach or park together and clean it up a bit.*
2. *Celebrate earth day; have dinner at home with her, "a la nude."*

Administrative Professionals Day / Week
-Celebrating Tips
Celebrate your good employees: give them their gifts and/or take them out to lunch, see if your wife can join you. Ask your wife to help you pick a gift for your secretary/assistant. (Definitely have your wife join you if you want to take your female staff out to eat.)

Arbor Day
Date varies from state to state from January to May
-Celebrating Tips
1. *Dedicate a forest, or a tree, in a park to your spouse or family.*
2. *To show your consideration and optimism for our planet, plant a tree with your mate and family.*

OTHER OBSERVANCES FOR THIS MONTH

- **Pesach / Passover** – March or April
- **Cancer Control Month**
- **Alcohol Awareness Month**
- **Patriots' Day**
- **Palm Sunday** – March or April
- **Good Friday** – March or April
- **Easter** – March or April
- **Patriot's Day**
- **Ascension Day** – This date varies by different faiths and religions.

May

Flower: Lily of the Valley, Lily

Birthstone: Emerald–*love, success*

Make this a Mother's Day Month.

-Celebrating Tips
1. If she is a mom: in the month of May, try to do as many of her chores as possible or hire a maid (of her choosing) to help out. This especially applies if she is a stay-at-home Mom.
2. Rent her dream car for the month/week/day, for her to drive.

Cinco de Mayo
-Celebrating Tips
1. Celebrate Cinco de Mayo. Learn about the Mexican culture. Go to a Mexican restaurant for dinner.
2. Have a Mexican style dinner party with mariachi band and all.

National Teachers Day / Teacher Appreciation Week
First Tuesday in May / First Full week in May
-Celebrating Tips
Great Teachers Make Great Schools… Don't forget the gifts for Teacher's Day; even a simple "thank you" card will be appreciated.

National Day of Prayer – 1st Thursday in May
-Celebrating Tips
1. Pray with the spouse/kids for the country, its leaders and your friends, etc.
2. Join your church, synagogue or community in a prayer service or event.

Mother's Day – 2nd Sunday in May
-Celebrating Tips
Wake her up with kisses, breakfast in bed, her favorite flowers and a gift. Carry out your celebrating plans for the day.

Nurses Day – May 12th
-Celebrating Tips
Don't forget the gifts for your favorite nurses and celebrate the good nurses in your local Hospital. You and your mate should treat them to lunch/dinner and gifts.

Police Week – Week in which May 15 occurs
-<u>Celebrating Tips</u>
Support your local police department.

Armed Forces Day – 3rd Saturday in May **"America Supports You"**
-<u>Celebrating Tips</u>
See how you can be a blessing to those who protect this Country.

Memorial Day – Last Monday in May
-<u>Celebrating Tips</u>
1. *Talk about what to do for Memorial Day weekend.*
2. Have a happy Memorial Day weekend!

National Safe Boating Week
-<u>Celebrating Tips</u>
If you own a boat, take the family boating. Or go to a lake in the park and play with a motorized toy boat, or go canoeing or paddle boat riding. You can also go boat window-shopping and pick out a boat that the family would love to own in the future.

ADDITIONAL OBSERVANCES FOR THIS MONTH

- **Lag B'Omer** – May
- **Shavu'ot** – May or June
- **Asian/Pacific American Heritage Month**
- **National Physical Fitness & Sports Month**
- **Steelmark Month**
- **Law day** – May 1st
- **Loyalty Day** – May 1st (display U.S. flag)
- **May Day** – May 1st – the Real Labor Day
- **Join Hands Day** – 1st Saturday in May
- **Peace officers Memorial Day** – 15th day of May
- **National Maritime Day** – 22nd Day of May
- **National Defense Transportation Day** – 3rd Friday in May
- **Peace Officers Memorial Day** – 15th day of May

(If you haven't done it yet, this is the time that you can start a Christmas savings account.)

June

*N*ational Rose Month

Roses date far back to pre-historic days. They are more than 33 million years old and have been used among friends and lovers to send all sorts of messages, and they are used for many reasons.

-Celebrating Tips
Give her roses every day or week this month. Send or personally give them to her, or place them where she will find them. If she works out of the home, send some to her at work. (Write in the note, card or love letter the meaning of the rose.)

ADDITIONAL OBSERVANCES FOR THIS MONTH

- **National Dairy Month**
- **Shavu'ot** – May or June, 50 days following Passover.
- **Ascension Day – Christian** – Observed in May or June
- **Atlantic Hurricane Season Begins** – June 1st
- **World Environment Day** – June 5th
-Celebrating Tips
Help your city organize a clean-up campaign, give a tree planting party or celebrate with a green concert and increase recycling awareness.
- **Philippines Independence Day** – June 11th
- **National Flag Week** – Week of June 14th – Display the flag of the United States.
- **Flag Day** – June 14th
- **Honor America Days** – June 14th thru July 4th
- **Father's Day** – 3rd Sunday in June
-Celebrating Tips
If you are a good Dad celebrate yourself: buy yourself that thing that you have been wanting.

- **Juneteenth** – 19th day of June. Also called "Freedom Day" or "Emancipation Day." It's the oldest known holiday to commemorate the end of slavery: June 19,1865.
- **Emancipation Day** – Date Varies in the United States, Puerto Rico and the Caribbean.
- **First Day of Summer** – June 20th or 21st Timed with the Summer Solstice.

-**Celebrating Tips**

1. *Surprise her by buying her a summer outfit or bathing suit that is of her taste.*

2. *Celebrate the first day of summer with a picnic theme dinner, including the short pants.*

3. *Stay up all night on Solstice Eve and welcome the rising Sun at dawn.*

- **St. Baptiste Day** – 24th day of June – French-Canadian
- **Ascension Day – Christian** – Observed in May or June
- **Helen Keller's Birthday** – June 27th
- **Paul Bunyan** – June 28th

Make plans for the 4th of July; take a long weekend or your vacation that week.

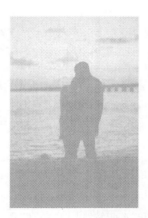

(Place a "Romantic" picture of the two of you here.)

July

Birthstone: Ruby – *contentment*

Tisha B'Av – July or August
Canada Day – July 1st (July 2nd if July 1st is on a Sunday)
Independence Day – July 4th
<u>-Celebrating Tips</u>
1. *If you do not have any plans to go away for the July 4th weekend, take July 4th off and have a beach party, invite family and friends.*
2. *Go ahead, take July 4th off along with her and go for a picnic or spend the day at your favorite hotel and enjoy the fire works at night. Flirt with her in a sexual way and make your own fireworks!*

Bastille Day – 14th day of July – French National Holiday
Parents' Day – 4th Sunday in July
…he who has a wise son delights in him. Pr. 23: 24b
<u>-Celebrating Tips</u>
1. *Invite the parents over for a cookout to celebrate Parent's Day.*
2. *Give them an award for being the best parents (plaque, medal or trophy).*

August

Tisha B'Av – July or August
Ramadan – 9th Month of the Muslim Calendar – August or September
Every year Islamic holidays happen earlier and they don't always occur in the same season.

Friendship Day – 1st Sunday in August
Honor your good friends and let them know that they are greatly valued.
<u>**-Celebrating Tips**</u>
1. *Get together with your friends and have a brunch party, hand out gifts or medals to acknowledge their wonderful contribution to your life.*
2. *Be a good neighbor.*

Assumption Day – 15th day of Aug – Christian

National Aviation Day – 19th day of August – Orville Wright's Birthday 1871

Women's Equality Day – August 26th
<u>**-Celebrating Tips**</u>
- *Help her to celebrate her rights.*

Make plans for Labor Day

NOTES/COMMENTS/JOURNAL

....

Keep a arecord of what worked, changes made or new ideas

September

Labor Day – 1st Monday in September
-Celebrating Tips
1. *Go away for the weekend or spend it doing something you both enjoy.*
2. Have a happy Labor Day weekend!

Ramadan – 9th Month of the Muslim Calendar – August or September
Every year Islamic holidays happen earlier and they don't always occur in the same season.

Islamic Eid ul-Fitr

Rosh Hashanah (Feast of Trumpets) – September
Jewish Holidays happen on a different day every year, and they begin in the fall starting with the celebration of the High Holy Days of Rosh Hashanah and Yom Kippur. The Jewish calendar coordinates with the rotation of the earth about its axis (a day), the revolution of the moon about the earth (a month), and the revolution of the earth about the sun (a year). All of the Jewish Holidays start at sundown the night before.

Yom Kippur – September - October

Grandparents Day – 1st Sunday after Labor Day in September
Honor your grandparents. Talk to your children about the wealth of information and character development that their grandparents can give. Grandparents can also celebrate their grandchildren and show them love. Grandparents Day is a day to further strengthen the spirit of love and respect for our elders.
-Celebrating Tips
1. *Have a family get-together. Play old family music; sing those old songs with grandpa and/or grandma, dance the old dances. Ask grandma to share her cooking recipes.*

2. *Let the grandparents tell the stories of their life, and how it was for them growing up.*
3. *Show the children and/or Grandchildren the old photographs in your family albums.*
4. *Put together a family tree photo album.*
5. *Talk about your family's ethnic or religious beliefs.*

Patriot Day – September 11, 2001
-Celebrating Tips
Take time out today to pray for the families and survivors of 9/11/01. Pray also for world peace and for God's protection over the U.S.A. and the world from terrorists.

National Hispanic Heritage Month – Sept. 15th – Oct. 15
-Celebrating Tips
1. *Celebrate with your local Hispanic community.*
2. *Sign up for Salsa classes this month as a couple.*
3. *Go visit a Spanish museum or Art gallery.*
4. *Celebrate Hispanic Heritage; go out to dinner at a Latin restaurant. Make sure that you dress sexy. Be very flirtatious in the way you talk and caress her. Tell her in Spanish: "Te vez muy linda." Translation: "You look beautiful." Say it with passion. (For more "foreign love talk" see Part seven, page 216.)*

Stepfamily Day – 16th day of September
-Celebrating Tips
If you are a stepfamily, go and do something fun and let each other know how much you love and appreciate each other.

Constitution Day & Week – September 17th

International Day Of Peace – 21st

Native American Day – 4th Friday in September
-Celebrating Tips
1. *Visit your local Native American museum or art gallery.*
2. *Celebrate with your local Native Americans.*
3. *Learn about the Native Americans.*
4. *Play along with her treat.*

First day of Autumn
-Celebrating Tips
Bring home an autumn bouquet.

Enjoy the Fall Season

*G*o on a hayride (hug and kiss)

....

*R*ent a cabin in the mountains for a long weekend

....

*T*ake a walk or a drive and enjoy the beautiful color changes

....

*I*f either of you enjoy the sport of hunting, go on a hunting trip

....

*M*ake out on a pile of fallen leaves, in a private
place at the park or in your backyard

Benilda Nya

October

Flower: Magnolia

Birthstone: Opal, Tourmaline–*hope*

National Hispanic Heritage Month Sept. 15th – Oct. 15th
-Celebrating Tips
1. Learn together about the Hispanic Heritage.
2. *CELEBRATE Hispanic month…*
Go to a costume shop and buy a Zorro mask or the complete outfit (keep it a secret). Take her out dancing at a Latin dance club, and put on your Latin lover charm (look & smell good). When you get back home, put on your Zorro mask/outfit; speak with your best Spanish accent, kiss her, tell her how much you desire her, in Spanish "Te Amo," "Te quiero," (translation: "I love you," "I want you"). "Tu eres mi tesoro," (translation: "You are my treasure"). "Mi reina," (translation: "My queen"). Then later, make your lovemaking "Muy Caliente" (very hot). (For more foreign "love talk," see Part seven, page 216 and 217.)

Yom Kippur – September – October

Sukkot – September – October

Shemi ni Atzeret – September – October

Simchat Torah – October

National Breast Cancer Month

National Disability Employment Awareness Month

Child Health Day – 1st Monday
-Celebrating Tips
Help your child to understand the benefits of taking care of their health.

National Children's Day – 8th
-Celebrating Tips
Show the children in your life how much you love and value them.

Leif Erikson Day – 9th
National School Lunch Week **(9-13)**
-Celebrating Tips
Call your kids' school, and see if there is anything you can do for "Lunch Week."

Columbus Day Observed – 2nd Monday, Display U.S. flag

Thanksgiving – Canada – 2nd Monday

White Cane Safety Day – 15th

National Forest Products Week **(15-21)**
-Celebrating Tips
If you have kids old enough, get with your mate & ask them to do a research on forest products.

National Boss Day – 16th
-Celebrating Tips
1. *Why don't you and your wife take your boss (yours and/or hers) and his/her significant other out to lunch or dinner?*
2. *Give your boss a gift.*
3. *Give a breakfast to honor your boss.*

Boss's Day

If you are "The Boss," make sure that you are a great boss. According to their expertise, pay them well. Be fair; encourage, praise and reward your employees (for a job well-done, an employee can get a spa day or financial bonus). Be concerned with their overall needs, and have a support system so that they will know your company is worth their loyalty, dedication and hard work.

Give your business or office a "happy" makeover. Find out what can make your employees happy at work, so that the business and production can increase. HAPPINESS = less stress, less sick time taken, better creativity, improved interactions with co-workers and clients, promotions and increased success and more profits. If possible, provide day care (for a small fee) on the premises. You can also help your employees release stress: make available a room with plants, a water fountain, floor mats,

CD player with relaxing music, a TV-video player where they can play yoga, tai chi or Qigong DVDs/videos to de-stress. A place where they can do deep breathing and stretching exercises for about fifteen minutes a day (it could be before the start of the day or some time in the middle of the workday). Don't allow eating lunch at the desk while working (that goes for the boss, also).

The lunch/break room should be nicely decorated (plants, water fountain) and well stocked. (Your employees should feel well cared for if you want them to perform great for you. At the same time, they need to know that you mean business and you need to run your company at its best.)

PLEASE, let your employees enjoy their day off and vacations, do not call them for anything. Also, do not micro-manage your people. If you need to, get rid of incompetent or lazy employees. Hire the right people even if it takes time to do so.

If you are the "employee," make sure that you are trustworthy, responsible and dedicated. Constantly increase the knowledge that concerns your duties and your professional goals. Skilled happy employees get promoted or asked to become a partner in the company.

Benilda Nya

A wise man's heart guides his mouth, and his lips
promote instruction. Proverbs 16: 23

Like the coolness of snow at harvest time is a trustworthy
messenger (employee) to those who send him; he refreshes
the spirit of his masters (employer). Proverbs 25: 13

Sweetest Day – 3rd Saturday
-Celebrating Tips
Give candy, flowers or gifts to the people in your life who are aged, sick, orphaned children, and the ones who are caring.

Mother-In-Law Day – 4th Sunday
-Celebrating Tips
Invite the in-laws (your parents and hers) out to brunch or dinner, if possible.

United Nations day – 24th

Halloween
-Celebrating Tips
Not everybody likes to celebrate Halloween, but you can make it fun and wholesome for your kids by having your own party without the scary costumes.

Throw a Romantic Costume Ball

Get together with your mate and pick a romantic era or romantic couples throughout history and have a "couples" costume party based on the way they dressed. Invite your friends, family, neighbors, business partners and co-workers.

Benilda Nya

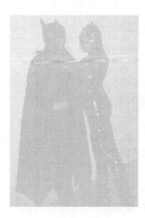

(Place a picture of both of you in a costume here.)

November

National American Indian Heritage Month

Good Nutrition Month

Aviation Month

Daylight-Saving Time Ends (set clocks back)

All Saints' Day – 1st

All Souls' Day – 2nd

Guy Fawkes Day – 5th - United Kingdom

Veteran's Day – 11th U.S. End WW1

Remembrance Day – 11th - Canada - End WW1 - 1918

Armistice Day – 11th - Europe - End WW1 - 1918

Thanksgiving Day – 3rd Thursday
-Celebrating Tips
1. *Help your wife with the preparations for Thanksgiving Day, or ask her how you can help.*
2. *Smile, be happy, and use your table etiquette; be a good host. Help her cleanup.*

Give Thanks

❤ Thanksgiving Day is what it is, "Thanksgiving." Make it a family affair by having your older kids prepare and read the story of the Pilgrims and the Indians. They could even wear costumes and make a little play out of it. If you do not have any kids but are having young nieces and nephews come over, have them read the "Thanksgiving story."

- **I**f the dinner is in your home, the thanksgiving prayer should go around the table starting at your left, as each person gives thanks for whom and for what they are thankful. It should end with you or your wife.

- **T**he carving of the turkey should be done by either you or your wife (who ever does it best), unless the grandfather has been the one to do it throughout the years, or any other person that you agree does a great job at carving the turkey.

Benilda Nya

Gobble Gobble

- **S**ome men take great pride in cooking the turkey, so if you are one of those men that can cook a delicious turkey, go ahead have your fun. If you would also like to help with any other cooking, baking and cleaning, that is great especially, if you and your wife are the ones having the families over to your house for the dinner.

- **F**ind a homeless shelter to help: whether you donate food or your time by stepping out earlier in the day to help serve. Share your blessings; feed the hungry.

- **P**lease don't let football be your reason for Thanksgiving Day. If you cannot miss your favorite team, either tape the game or talk it over with your wife and find the perfect time to serve dinner, so that your family can have your undivided attention.

Benilda Nya

Take Joy in the Holidays

According to your religious and family traditions, make sure that you are a vital part of all the festivities. Make it one of the happiest and fun times in your home. This will not only give you points with her, but it will also be a good example and support for your children.

Benilda Nya

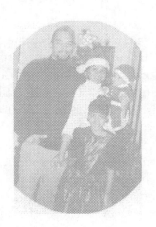

(Place a holiday family picture here.)

December

Flower: Hibiscus, Holly, Poinsettia

Birthstone: Turquoise, Zircon - *prosperity*

-Celebrating Tips
Build a snowman together.

-Celebrating Tips
1. *Buy yourself a sexy Santa Claus outfit to play her "Santa" on Christmas Eve or Day.*
2. *Give her money to go Christmas shopping.*
3. *Help her wrap the Christmas gifts, drink some eggnog, listen to Christmas songs, laugh, be happy.*

Ashura – December or January - This Islamic holiday is observed on the 10th of Muharram, the first month of the Islamic year.

Hanukkah – December, every few years in November

AIDS Awareness Day – 1st
-Celebrating Tips
Talk to your older children about the danger of HIV and AIDS.

Nat'l Pearl Harbor Remembrance Day – 7th

Human Rights Day – 10th

Wright Brother's Day – 17th
-Celebrating Tips
Play Captain and Co-pilot.

Pan American Aviation Day – 17th
-Celebrating Tips
Play Passenger and Flight Attendant.
Forefather's Day – 21st

First Day of Winter – 21st or 22nd - The shortest day of the year
-Celebrating Tips
1. *Go shopping for matching winter outfits.*
2. *Take her to the park for a carriage ride. Bring along two cups and a thermos filled with hot chocolate and marshmallows. Serve it while riding to keep warm.*

National Regifting Day – Thursday before Christmas

Christmas Eve – 24th
-Celebrating Tips
Be a "good" Santa.

Merry Christmas!

**Gather up those Christmas lists; time to withdraw
from that Christmas account, and start shopping.**

....

If you have kids (and they can enjoy helping you choose the gifts), take
them with you and your wife to do the Christmas shopping for your
family, friends, Minister/Pastor/Rabbi/Priest, boss and co-workers.

....

**Have a budget and stick to it. Instead of buying a gift for each
person in a family, you can buy one thing that every-body can enjoy.**

....

If your wife's or kids' list is longer than your budget,
ask them to prioritize (1-5, five being the least desirable).
But do not give away the element of surprise.

....

**For Christmas you can give her a gift a day for
the twelve Days of Christmas. Or for Hanukkah:
give her one for each of the eight days.**

....

Help each other to wrap the gifts, and play
Christmas songs and drink some eggnog.

Benilda Nya

Join in the Reindeer games

Play Christmas music while having dinner.

. . . .

Go for a drive or walk to see the decorated homes and streets.

. . . .

If you have children or teens that are a part of their school, church or community Christmas play, make sure that you go with your wife to see them perform.

. . . .

Enjoy taking your wife or the whole family to see a Christmas play or movie. Or surprise them with tickets for them to go if you can't make it.

. . . .

Take your wife/family to a Christmas amusement park; get on the rides with her/them; act silly, laugh, eat and have fun.

. . . .

Get together with your friends, neighbors and/ or family, and give a fun Christmas party.

Benilda Nya

Oh, Christmas Tree

*S*hop for the Christmas tree together, or surprise her with it.

....

*H*elp with the decorating of the tree.

....

If your thing is decorating the house inside and/or outside, have fun. Let her know if you need her help or input.

....

*D*on't forget to hang the mistletoe, and kiss her under it.

Benilda Nya

Pleasing Her During the Holidays

If you have not yet told her how beautiful the house looks, thanked her for the delicious cookies/cake or food, & told her how much you appreciate her helping you to pick out the gifts for your family, friends, co-workers, boss, secretary or friends; this will be a good time to do so.

....

*H*ave you complimented her on how beautiful she looks?

....

If you have kids old enough to appreciate a compliment, make sure that you thank them for their good behavior. If they helped to decorate and keep the house clean, thank them for helping, and if they are wearing something that looks great; tell them.

....

*A*sk if she needs help with anything, or if she needs anything from the store. Be attentive to her needs during the holiday season to help ease the load.

Benilda Nya

Christmas Day – 25th
Merry Christmas!
<u>**-Celebrating Tips**</u>
Be a good example of the Christmas spirit; be joyful and thankful in everything.

Kwanzaa – December 26th thru Jan. 1st

Boxing Day – 26th - Canada

New Year's Eve – 31st
Have a Happy and Prosperous New Year, full of Romance!

Part Four

Flowers and Their Meaning

The Meaning Of Color For Flowers

When you give flowers or buy flowers for yourself, you can choose the mood and ambiance you want to create as well as the meaning and message you want to send. Yes, by simply choosing the kind of flower and the color(s) you can produce the environment you want to establish for yourself and others.

With the information about flowers in this section, you can be as creative and purposeful as you would like to be. When sending flowers to some one, add in the meaning on the card or letter so that they can be inspired and appreciate the flowers even more.

Purposeful Color

VIOLET – analogous with royalty, aristocracy, a symbol of faith and spirituality; it's energizing. Tell the recipient that they are extraordinary

BLUE – can improve your enthusiasm, it helps to heighten creativity, its soothing and it invites in a peaceful environment. Blue flowers impart a calm solution to our overly stressed lives and schedules

RED – represents love, vitality, passion & desire

ORANGE – the color of friendship, represents progress and sincerity, increase

YELLOW – admiration, gratefulness, provision, wisdom, lucidity, loyalty

INDIGO – perfect for people who multi-task/very busy people. Get in touch with deep feelings and show them. Helps to take it down a notch, increase on quality time

The Meaning Of Color For Roses

❤ **Red Roses:** "I love you." Passionate love. Romantic love. Admiration. Valor.

❤ **White Roses:** Innocence. Secrecy and silence. "I am worthy of you." Purity. Charm. Reverence. Humility. Spiritual love. "You are heavenly." Youthfulness.

❤ **Bridal White:** Happy love.

❤ **Yellow:** Joy. Gladness. Friendship. Devotion. Try to care. Welcome back. Remember me. Infidelity and jealousy.

❤ **Coral Roses:** Enthusiasm. Desire.

❤ **Orange:** Fascination. You are my secret love.

❤ **Light Peach:** Modesty of friendship.

❤ **Light Pink:** Grace. Gentility. Admiration. Sympathy.

❤ **Dark pink:** Say "Thank you." Appreciation. Gratitude.

❤ **Pink:** Perfect happiness. Love. "Thank you." Grace. Admiration.

❤ **Deep Burgundy:** "Unconscious beauty." Mourning.

❤ **Pale colored Roses:** Signify friendship.

❤ **Lavender:** Mean love at first sight.

❤ **Champagne:** You are tender and loving.

❤ **Red and White Together:** signify unity.

❤ **White and Purple Together:** Symbolic representations of purity and passion.

❤ **Pink and White:** I love you still and always will.

❤ **Yellow and Orange Together:** Passionate thoughts.

❤ **Red and Yellow Together:** Are an expression of congratulations or happy feelings.

❤ **Rose (tea):** I'll always remember you.

❤ **Rose (Christmas):** Peace and tranquility.

❤ **Rose (musk cluster):** Capricious beauty.

❤ **Rose (hibiscus):** Delicate beauty.

❤ **Black Rose:** You are my obsession. Death.

❤ **Assorted Color Roses Together:** You're everything to me.

❤ **A Crown made of Roses:** Signifies reward of merit or virtue.

When giving the flowers, use the meaning of it as part of the poem, love letter or note; you can also give the flowers along with her favorite stuffed animal, chocolates, balloons, jewelry, or a CD of her favorite music.

The Story of Roses

- ❤ **Thornless Rose:** Love at first sight.
- ❤ **Long Stemmed Rose:** "I will remember you always."
- ❤ **Short Stemmed Rose:** Sweetheart. Girlhood.
- ❤ **Rosebud:** Beauty and youth. A heart innocent of love.
- ❤ **Rosebud (white):** Girlhood; too young to love.
- ❤ **Rosebud (red):** Pure and lovely.
- ❤ **Rosebud (moss):** Confessions of love.
- ❤ **A Single Rose:** Any color – "I appreciate you."
- ❤ **A Single Rose:** Red in full bloom – "My love for you is unchanged," or "I still love you."
- ❤ **2 Roses:** Taped or wired together to form a single stem signal an engagement or coming marriage.
- ❤ **2 Roses:** We both feel the same deep love. We share the same feelings.
- ❤ **3 Roses:** "I love you."
- ❤ **A full blown Rose placed over two buds:** Secrecy.
- ❤ **6 Roses:** "I want to be yours."
- ❤ **7 Roses:** "I'm head over heels in love with you."
- ❤ **9 Roses:** "We'll be together for ever." Eternal love.
- ❤ **10 Roses:** "You are perfect."
- ❤ **11 Roses:** "You are the one I cherish." "You are my treasured one."
- ❤ **12 Roses:** "I want you to be mine!" Pleasurable combination. Combined likeness.
- ❤ **13 Roses:** "We are for ever friends." Secret admirer.
- ❤ **15 Roses:** "I apologize." "I'm truly sorry."
- ❤ **20 Roses:** "My feelings towards you are sincere."
- ❤ **21 Roses:** "I'm totally committed to you." "I'm dedicated to you."
- ❤ **24 Roses:** Keep me lovingly in your mind, all the time. "I cannot get you out of my mind." "Forever yours."
- ❤ **25 Roses:** "Well done." "Bravo." "Congratulations."
- ❤ **33 Roses:** "My love for you is INTENSE." Affection.
- ❤ **36 Roses:** "Reminiscing our romantic time together." I am experiencing romantic affections towards you every time you come near me.
- ❤ **40 Roses:** "My love for you is genuine."
- ❤ **44 Roses:** My vow to you is faithful and consistent. Unchangeable pledge.

- **50 Roses:** This is "Regretless/Unconditional Love."
- **56 Roses:** My darling.
- **66 Roses:** Successful love affair.
- **99 Roses:** "I will love you all the days of my life." Love with understanding makes love eternal.
- **100 Roses:** The most pleasurable marriage of the century. We are dedicated to each other forever.
- **101 Roses:** "There is no one else for me but you." Totally committed to you.
- **108 Roses:** "Will you marry me." "Will you take my hand in holy matrimony?"
- **111 Roses:** Endless love.
- **123 Roses:** Free love.
- **144 Roses:** I love you day and night, forever.
- **365 Roses:** Thinking of you every day. I love you each and every day.
- **999 Roses:** "I will love you 'till the end of time."
- **1001 Roses:** Faithful love. 'Till forever.
- **Rose leaves:** Long for. Hope.

More Flowers

A

Amaranth	Immortal Love
Amaryllis	Beauty; Dramatic; Pride
Anthurium	Hospitality
Aster	Elegance; Variety; Symbol of Love; Daintiness, Contentment
Azalea	Temperance; First love; Romance; Fragile Passion; Love

B

Baby's Breath	Innocence
Bamboo	Steadfastness; Strength; Loyalty
Begonia	Beware; Fanciful Nature; Be Cordial; Deep thoughts
Bird of Paradise	Magnificence; Freedom; Good Perspective; Given at ninth wedding anniversary

C

Cactus	Endurance; Warmth
Carnation, General	Fascination; Woman; Divine Love
Carnation, Pink	I'll Never Forget You; Motherly Love; Gratitude
Carnation, Red	My Heart Aches For You; Admiration; I Hold You in High Esteem; Respect; Deep Love, Friendship
Carnation, Purple	Capriciousness
Carnation, Solid Color	Yes
Carnation, Striped	No; Refusal; Sorry, I Can't Be With You; Wish I Could Be With You
Carnation, White	Sweet and Lovely; Innocence; Pure Love; Woman's Good Luck Gift
Carnation, Yellow	You Have Disappointed Me; Rejection; The 13th wedding anniversary flower
Chrysanthemum	(in general) Cheerfulness; Optimism; Rest; Truth; Long Life; joy; You are a Wonderful Friend

Chrysanthemum, Red	I Love you
Chrysanthemum, White	Loyal love, Truthfulness
Chrysanthemum, Yellow	Slighted Love; Secret Admirer; Chivalry
Cyclamen	Resignation; Good-bye

D

Daffodil	Chivalry; Rebirth; New beginnings; Regard; Unrequited Love; You're the Only One; Given for the 10th wedding anniversary
Daisy	Love that conquers all; Innocence; Loyal Love; I'll keep your secret; Purity; Gentleness; Given for the fifth wedding anniversary
Daisy, Red	Joy
Daisy, White	Innocence; Truth
Daisy, Yellow	I will try hard to earn your Love
Gerbera Daisy	Cheerfulness
Dandelion	Faithfulness; Happiness; Wishes come True; Oracle of Time and Love

E

Eucalyptus	Protection

F

Fern	Sincerity; Magic; Fascination; Confidence; Shelter
Fern, Maidenhair	Secret bond of love
Freesia	Innocence; Thoughtfulness; Spirited
Fir	Time
Forget-Me-Not	True Love; Memories; Remember me forever
Forsythia	Anticipation
Fuschia	Amiability; Taste; Given for third wedding anniversary

G

Gardenia	Joy; My Secret Love; You are lovely

Gladiolus	Strength of Character; I am really Sincere; Flower of the gladiators
Gloxinia	Love at First Sight

H

Heather, Pink	"Good Luck"
Heather, Purple	Admiration; Beauty and Solitude
Heather, White	Protection; Wishes Will Come True
Hibiscus	Delicate Beauty
Holly	Domestic Happiness
Hyacinth, General	Games and Sports; dedicated to Apollo
Hyacinth, Blue	Constancy; Predictability; Reliable
Hyacinth, Purple	I am Sorry; Please Forgive me; Sorrow
Hyacinth, Red or Pink	Play
Hyacinth, White	Loveliness; I Will Pray for You
Hyacinth, Yellow	Jealousy
Hydrangea	Thank You for Understanding; Heartlessness

I

Iris	Faith; Wisdom; Valor; Your Friendship means so much to me; My Compliments; Fleur-de-lis; Emblem of France; Passion; Inspiration; Given for 25th wedding anniversary
Iris White	Purity
Iris Blue	Faith; Hope
Iris Yellow	Passion
Iris Purple	Wisdom; Compliments
Ivy	Fidelity; Friendship; Wedded Love; Affection; Marriage

J

Jasmine	Amiability; attracts wealth; Grace & Elegance
Jasmine, Red	Folly; Glee
Jasmine, Yellow	Timidity; Modesty

Jasmine Spanish	Sensuality
Jonquil	Love Me; Affection Returned; Violent Desire/ Sympathy

L

Larkspur	Open heart; Beautiful spirit
Larkspur, Pink	Fickleness
Larkspur, Purple	First love; Sweet Disposition
Larkspur, White	Joyful; Happy-go Lucky
Lavender	Success; Luck; Happiness; Constancy; Distrust
Lilac	Youthful; Confidence; Humility
Lilac, Mauve	"Do you still Love me?"
Lilac, Pink	Youth; Acceptance
Lilac, Purple	You are my first Love
Lilac, White	"My first Dream of Love"
Lily	Majesty; Wealth; Pride; Innocence; Purity
Lily, Calla	Majestic Beauty; I am in Heaven When I'm With You; Associated with the sixth wedding anniversary
Lily, Casablanca	Celebration
Lily, Day	Coquetry; Chinese Emblem for Mother
Lily, Orange	Flame; I burn for you; Hatred; Disdain
Lily, Pink	Youth and Acceptance; Romantic
Lily, Stargazer	I See Heaven in Your Eyes
Lily, Tiger	Wealth; Pride
Lily, White	Majesty; Purity; Virginity; It's heavenly to be with you; My love is pure and innocent
Lily, Yellow	Live for the Moment; I'm Walking on Air
Lily- Of -The- Valley	Humility; Sweetness; Return to Happiness; Tears of the Virgin Mary; You've Made My Life Complete
Lotus	Mystery and Truth

M

Magnolia	Dignity; Nobility; Splendid Beauty
Marigold	Desire for riches; Sacred Affection; Cruelty; Grief; Jealousy

Mistletoe	Kiss me; Affection; To Surmount Difficulties; Sacred Plant of India
Myrtle	Love; Mirth; Joy; Hebrew Emblem of Marriage
Myrrh	Gladness

N

Narcissus	Egotism; Formality; Stay as Sweet as You Are

O

Orchid	Love; Rare Beauty; Beautiful lady; Refinement, Magnificence; Chinese symbol for many children; Given at the 28th wedding anniversary; long life

P

Palm leaves	Victory and Success
Pansy	Thoughtful Recollection of you, Loyalty; Symbolic of the Trinity because of their three colors; Can be given at the first wedding anniversary
Poinsettia	"Be of Good Cheer"
Poppy, General	Imagination; Dreaminess; Eternal Sleep; Ninth wedding anniversary
Poppy, Oriental	Silence is Golden
Poppy, Red	Pleasure; Consolation
Poppy, Scarlet	Extravagance
Poppy, White	Consolation; Tranquility
Poppy, Yellow	Wealth; Success
Primrose	Satisfaction; Happiness; Young Love; I cannot live with out You

S

Snowdrop	Hope
Sunflower	Homage and Devotion
Sweet Pea	Departure; Blissful Pleasure; Lasting Pleasure; Thank You for a Lovely Time; Shyness

T

Tulip	Symbol of The Perfect Lover; Flower Emblem of Holland
Tulip, Red	Believe Me; Declaration of Love
Tulip, Variegated	Beautiful Eyes
Tulip, Yellow	There's Sunshine in your Smile; I am hopelessly in Love
Tulip, Cream	I will Love you forever

V

Violet	Modesty; Virtue; Demureness; Faithfulness; Given for fiftieth wedding anniversary; Simplicity
Violet, Yellow	I Love My Country
Violet, Purple	Blue love; Thoughts of you
Violet, Blue	Watchfulness; Faithfulness; I'll always be true
Violet, White	Let's take a chance

W

Water Lily	Eloquence and Persuasion; Purity of Heart
Wisteria	Welcome

X

Xeranthemum	Cheerfulness under adverse conditions

Y

Yarrow	Health-giving; Sorrow

Z

Zinnia	Thinking of Friends not Present
Zinnia, Pink	Eternal Fondness
Zinnia, White	Goodness
Zinnia, Yellow	Daily Remembrance
Zinnia, Scarlet	Constancy

Part Five

More of Her Favorite Things

Her Favorite Romantic Songs

Name	Artist	Name	Artist

Her Favorite Boogie Songs

Name	Artist	Name	Artist

Her Favorite Restaurants

Steakhouse-Asian-Sushi-Caribbean-Latin-Mexican-Italian-
Middle Eastern-European-Bar & Bistro-Seafood-Buffet-Barbeque-
Sandwiches & Subs-Soup & Salad-Café-Deli-Sports Café/
Bar-Pizza-Health Food-Fast Food-Breakfast-Lunch-Gourmet-
Bakery-Takeout-Ice Cream Shop-Smoothie-Vegetarian

Name/Type	Location	Tel.

Her Favorite Theatres

Movie-Playhouse-Performing Arts-Arena-Concert Hall-Stadium

Name/Type	Location	Tel.

*H*er Favorite Supermarket &Pharmacy

Name/Type   Location   Tel.

_____

_____

_____

*H*er Favorite Household Cleaning Brands

Laundry Detergent:_____

Fabric Softener:_____

Bleach:_____

Disinfectant:_____

Glass Cleaner:_____ **All Purpose Cleaner:**_____

Floor:_____

Bathroom:_____

Kitchen: Dishwashing:_____

Other:_____

*H*er Favorite Food Brands

Type   Brand   Type   Brand

_____

_____

_____

_____

*H*er Favorite Personal Hygiene Brands

Type   **Brand**

_____

_____

_____

*H*er Favorite Bedding Brands

Thread Count:_____Bed Size:_____Mattress Type:_____

Circle Her Favorite Styles: Traditional - Casual - Modern - Country - Romantic

Favorite Colors:_____

Circle Her Favorites: Bed Spread - Comforter - Duvet Cover - Quilt - Blanket **Other:**_____

Pillow Size(s): Standard - King_____

Filling: Goose Down - Organic - Down Alternative_____

Decorative/Accent Pillows:_____

Fabrics: Cotton - Cotton Jersey - Egyptian Cotton - Flannel - Silky Satin Cotton Sateen - Organic **Other:**_____

Fabric Styles: Solid Colors - Stripes - Dots - Floral Prints - Lace - Pattern Animal Prints - Embroidered - Bordered

Designers:_____

Store Brands:_____

Organic Brands:_____

H̃er Favorite Parks & Recreation

Name/Type	Location	Tel.

H̃er Favorite Area Attractions

Museums-Zoo-Library-Planetarium & Observatory-Seaquarium
Botanical Garden-Beach-Art Gallery

Name/Type	Location	Tel.

H̃er Favorite Airports

Name/Type	Location	Tel.

H̃er Favorite Airlines

Name/Type	Location	Tel.

*H*er Favorite Cruise Line

Name/Type   Location   Tel.

_____

_____

_____

*H*er Favorite Electronic Brands

Name/Type   Location   Tel.

_____

_____

_____

_____

*H*er Favorite Appliance Brands

Name/Type   Location   Tel.

_____

_____

_____

_____

Part Six

Birthdays, Anniversaries, Contacts and Notes

Birthdays and Anniversaries

Date	Name	Occasion

Special People & Contacts

Name: _____

Address: _____

Telephone: _____ Email: _____

Name: _____

Address: _____

Telephone: _____ Email: _____

Name: _____

Address: _____

Telephone: _____ Email: _____

Name: _____

Address: _____

Telephone: _____ Email: _____

Name: _____

Address: _____

Telephone: _____ Email: _____

Name: _____

Address: _____

Telephone: _____ Email: _____

Special People & Contacts

Name:

Address:

Telephone: Email:

Name:

Address:

Telephone: Email:

Name:

Address:

Telephone: Email:

Name:

Address:

Telephone: Email:

Name:

Address:

Telephone: Email:

Name:

Address:

Telephone: Email:

Special People & Contacts

Name: _____

Address: _____

Telephone: _____ Email: _____

Name: _____

Address: _____

Telephone: _____ Email: _____

Name: _____

Address: _____

Telephone: _____ Email: _____

Name: _____

Address: _____

Telephone: _____ Email: _____

Name: _____

Address: _____

Telephone: _____ Email: _____

Name: _____

Address: _____

Telephone: _____ Email: _____

Notes

Notes

Notes

Part Seven

Fanning the Flames of Romance

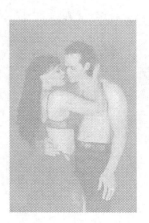

(Place a "sexy" picture here of the two of you.)

To fan the flames of romance...
Give each other sweet or sexy pet names

My Pleasure Garden

My Vision of Loveliness

My Lovely Desert Flower

My Lily of the Valleys

My Exotic Flower

Passion Puff

Sexy Mama

Angel Love

My Honey Bun

Gata (Beautiful Woman

Querida (Spanish - loved)

Amore Mio (Italian: my love)

Mi Vida (Spanish: my Life)

My One and Only Love

Dark and Lovely

My Beloved

My Darling

Bombshell

Baby Doll

My Queen

Sugar Nip

Sunflower

Sweet or Sexy Expressions
In other languages

English	French	Pronunciation
- My Love =	Mon Amour	Mon Nah-Moor
- My Life =	Ma Vie	Mah Vee
- Kiss Me! =	Embrasse - Moil!	Ahn-Brah S Mwah
- Yes =	Oui	Wee
- Please =	Sil vous plait	Seel Voo Ple
- Thank you =	Merci	Mer-See
- Hello =	Bonjour	Bon Zhoor
- I'm sorry =	Je suis de sole	Zhuh Swee Da-Sola
- Good-bye =	Au Revoir	O Ruh-Vwahr
- Good morning =	Bonjour	Bon Zhoor
- Good night =	Bonne Nuit	Buhn Nwee
- With pleasure! =	Avec plaisir!	Ah-ve K Pla-Zeer
- Well Done! =	Bravo!	Brah-Vo

English	Italian	Pronunciation
- My Love =	Amore Mio	Ah-mo-re mee-o
- My Life =	Vita Mia	Vee-tah mee-ah
- Kiss Me! =	Baciami!	Bah-chah-mee
- Come Here! =	Venga qui	Ven-gah kwee
- With Pleasure! =	Con piacere!	Kon pee-ah-che-re

- Farewell My Love! =   Addio Amore Mio!-------Ahd-dee-oh ah-moh-re mee-oh

- Perfect =   Perfetto--------------------------------Pehr-feht-toh

- Hello & Good-bye =   Ciao-------------------------------------Chah-oh

- Spicy =   Piccante-------------------------------Peek-kahn-teh

- Good =   Buono--------------------------------Boo-oh-noh

English	*Portuguese*	*Pronunciation*
- Beautiful Woman =	Gata------------------------------------	Gah-tah
- Handsome Man =	Gato------------------------------------	Gah-toh
- Let's Get To It =	Vamos la-----------------------------	Vah-mooz lah

English	*Spanish*	*Pronunciation*
- Beautiful (F) =	Bella------------------------------------	Bveh-yah
- Beautiful (M) =	Bello------------------------------------	Bveh-yoh
- Yes =	Si--------------------------------------	See
- Hello =	Hola------------------------------------	O-lah
- Good-bye =	Adios-----------------------------------	Ah-dee-os
- Kiss Me! =	Besame!---------------------------------	Be-sah-me
- My Life =	Mi Vida---------------------------------	Mee vee-dah
- My Love =	Mi Amor---------------------------------	Mee ah-mor
- Thank You =	Gracias---------------------------------	Grah-see-ahs

"*I Love You*"
In other languages

LANGUAGE	I LOVE YOU
1 - Arabic	Ana Behiback (to a male)
	Ana Behibek (to a female)
2 - Canadian	Sh'teme
3 - Chinese	Wo le Ni (Mandarin)
	Ngo oiy Ney a (Cantonese)
4 - Cherokee	Gvgeyuhi
5 - Czech	Miluji Te
6 - Danish	Jeg Elsker Dig
7 - Dutch	Ik Hou Van Jou
8 - Filipino	Mahal Kita
9 - French	Je T'aime, Je T'adore
10- German	Ich Liebe Dich
11- Greek	Saghapo (inf), Ssaghapo (frm)
12- Hebrew	Ani Ohev Otach (to female)
	Ani Ohevet Otcha (to male)
13- Hindi	Mai tumse Pyar karta hoon (to female)
	Mai tumse Pyar karti hoon (to male)
14- Indonesian	Saya mencintaimu
15- Irish	Graimthu
16- Italian	Ti Amo
17- Japanese	Kimi O Ai Shiteru
18- Korean	Sarang hac
19- Portuguese	Eu Te Amo
20- Russian	ja teb'a l'ubl'u
21- Spanish	Te Amo, Te Quiero
22- Swahili	Ninaku Penda
23- Swedish	Jag A'Lskar Dig
24- Zulu	Ngiyakuthanda!

FILL IN THE ACTIVITY THAT YOU WANT <u>YOUR SPOUSE TO DO</u>

(Use your best handwriting.)
Make plenty of copies in different types of papers and colors.

Request For Pleasure & Excitement

Request: _____

_____

Date: _____ Time: _____

Place: _____

FILL IN THE ACTIVITY THAT <u>YOU WANT TO</u> DO FOR YOUR SPOUSE

This Voucher Is Good For One Event

I will... _____

_____

Date: _____ Time: _____

FILL IN THE ACTIVITY THAT YOU WANT <u>YOUR SPOUSE TO DO</u>

(Use your best handwriting.)
Make plenty of copies in different types of papers and colors.

Request For Pleasure & Excitement

Request: _____

_____

Date: _____ *Time*: _____

Place: _____

FILL IN THE ACTIVITY THAT <u>YOU WANT TO</u> DO FOR YOUR SPOUSE

This Voucher Is Good For One Event

I Will... _____

_____

Date: _____ *Time*: _____

FILL IN THE ACTIVITY THAT YOU WANT <u>YOUR SPOUSE TO DO</u>

(Use your best handwriting.)
Make plenty of copies in different types of papers and colors.

Request For Pleasure & Excitement

Request: _____

_____

Date: _____ *Time:* _____

Place: _____

FILL IN THE ACTIVITY THAT <u>YOU WANT TO</u> DO FOR YOUR SPOUSE

This Voucher Is Good For One Event

I will... _____

_____

Date: _____ *Time:* _____

FILL IN THE ACTIVITY THAT YOU WANT <u>YOUR SPOUSE TO DO</u>

(Use your best handwriting.)
Make plenty of copies in different types of papers and colors.

Request For Pleasure & Excitement

Request: _____

_____

Date: _____ Time: _____

Place: _____

FILL IN THE ACTIVITY THAT <u>YOU WANT TO</u> DO FOR YOUR SPOUSE

This Voucher Is Good For One Event

I will... _____

_____

Date: _____ Time: _____

As A Man Thinks In His Heart, So Is He

Proverbs 23:7

Our life is what our thoughts make it.

– Marcus Aurelius

A man will find that as he alters his thoughts toward things, and other people, things and other people will alter towards him.

– James Allen

We are the sum total of what our thoughts are!!!

Wishing you good thoughts & a Life Filled With "Romance."

Benilda Nya

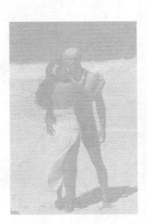

(Place one of your favorite pictures here of the two of you.)